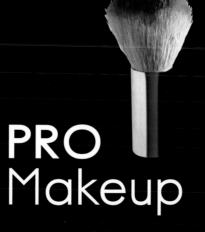

PRO
Makeup

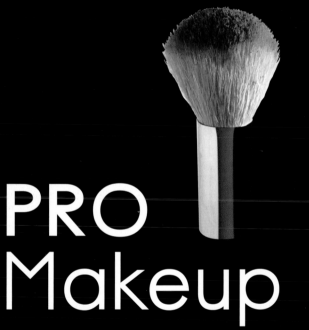

PRO
Makeup

Salon secrets of the professionals

Kit Spencer

FIREFLY BOOKS

A FIREFLY BOOK

Published by Firefly Books Ltd. 2009
Copyright © 2009 Quintet Publishing

First printing 2009

Publisher Cataloging-in-Publication Data (U.S.)

Spencer, Kit.
    PRO Makeup: Salon secrets of the professionals/Kit Spencer.
Includes index.
Summary: A complete guide to the skills, beauty secrets, and tricks essential to creating flawless makeup, either for daily wear or for special occasions. Step-by-step instructions and advice for all different skin tones, shapes and ages.
ISBN-13: 978-1-55407-477-8
ISBN-10: 1-55407-477-0
1. Cosmetics. 2. Beauty, Personal. I. Title.
646.7/26 dc22   RA778.S646 2009

Library and Archives Canada Cataloging in Publication
A CIP record for this book is available from Library and Archives Canada.

Published in the United States by
Firefly Books (U.S.) Inc.
P.O. Box 1338, Ellicott Station
Buffalo, New York 14205

Published in Canada by
Firefly Books Ltd.
66 Leek Crescent
Richmond Hill, Ontario L4B 1H1

Conceived, designed, and produced by
Quintet Publishing Limited
6 Blundell Street
London N7 9BH, UK

Project Editor: Asha Savjani
Editorial Assistant: Tanya Laughton
Photographer: Martin Norris
Designer: Anna Gatt
Illustrator: Bernard Chau
Art Director: Michael Charles
Managing Editor: Donna Gregory
Publisher: James Tavendale

Printed in China

CONTENTS

ABOUT THIS BOOK

This book will help you develop your own makeup routine. The author's sound practical advice, tips, and tricks make doing your own makeup, as well as applying makeup to others, easy. You will learn how to make the most of your unique skin type and tone combination, giving you the confidence and skills needed to try new styles.

➲ Detailed photography and annotations explain the essential equipment of your makeup bag as well as the more advanced tools you may wish to experiment with.
See pages 38–41.

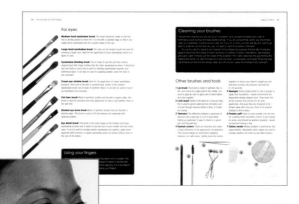

⬅ The essential techniques, such as applying foundation, are covered in detail. See pages 36–125.

➲ Once the fundamental techniques of good makeup have been established, the author explains how to develop different looks. At every stage variations are shown; they are a guide to how these looks transfer to different skin types and tones, as well as on women of different ages. See pages 126–93.

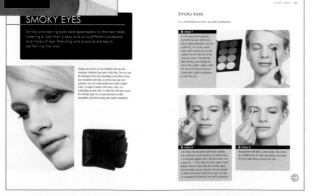

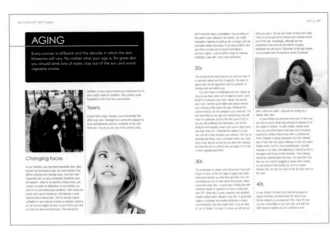

⬅ The various effects of aging are explained in relation to the skin, and advice is given on how to care for older skin effectively, as well as how to develop age-appropriate looks. See pages 122–4.

➡ Detailed and extensive step-by-step instructions for applying your own or another's bridal makeup. The various considerations for the bride-to-be are discussed at length, and advice is given for brides who want to look good from a distance without overwhelming those standing close by. Includes practical considerations for mother-in-laws and bridesmaids. See pages 182–93.

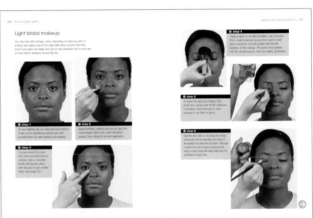

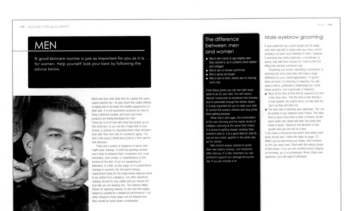

⬅ This last chapter covers teaching men to care for their skin and how to look good for a special occasion, as well as teaching you how to apply washable facepaints to children and prepare your friends for a costume party. See pages 194–245.

INTRODUCTION

I have been a makeup artist for over 10 years. During this time I have worked on every combination of face shape, skin tone, and age of woman possible. It still surprizes me how unconfident the majority of women feel about choosing and applying their own makeup. Makeup is not only exciting and creative, but it also has an amazingly empowering quality. It is not difficult or time-consuming to apply natural, daytime or evening makeup when you know how to do it properly. It is right to feel frustrated that you wear the same shade of lipstick day and night, whether you're shopping for groceries or going to a party. Now is the time to update your makeup techniques, give your makeup bag an overhaul, start looking at new colors, and invest in decent brushes.

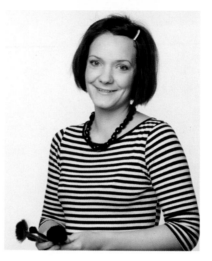

Makeup can make you look and feel better. Its purpose is to enhance your face and features, not disguise them. Makeup, when applied well, blends flawlessly into the skin tone. There are no hard edges, and all the features are balanced. All the individual elements—eyes, lips, and cheeks—work with each other. Badly applied makeup sits on the surface of the skin, looks patchy, and is aging. The key to achieving success is learning how to apply makeup properly, starting with the basics such as selecting and applying foundation, using concealer, and contouring. Once you've mastered the basics, you can achieve whatever look you desire, because you'll have the confidence to start experimenting.

About this book

As a professional you must have the skills to apply makeup to anyone and everyone. As an individual, you just need the knowledge and skills to apply makeup to the one face you know the best—your own. Through teaching and observing women doing their own makeup, I know the common pitfalls and mistakes that women encounter, and I will teach you how to avoid them, using clear step-by-step instructions and pictures of real women.

This book will help you develop a makeup routine that can be easily adapted to whatever time you have available, whether it is 10 minutes in the morning or 30 minutes before a party or big event. By breaking your routine down into separate elements such as base, blush, mascara, and eye looks, you should be able to pick and choose elements to fit the time available. The more you practice, the quicker you will get. The skills required and the basic steps followed for applying natural eye makeup and a dramatic smoky eye, for example, are the same. Sometimes even the same colors are used, but the intensity of

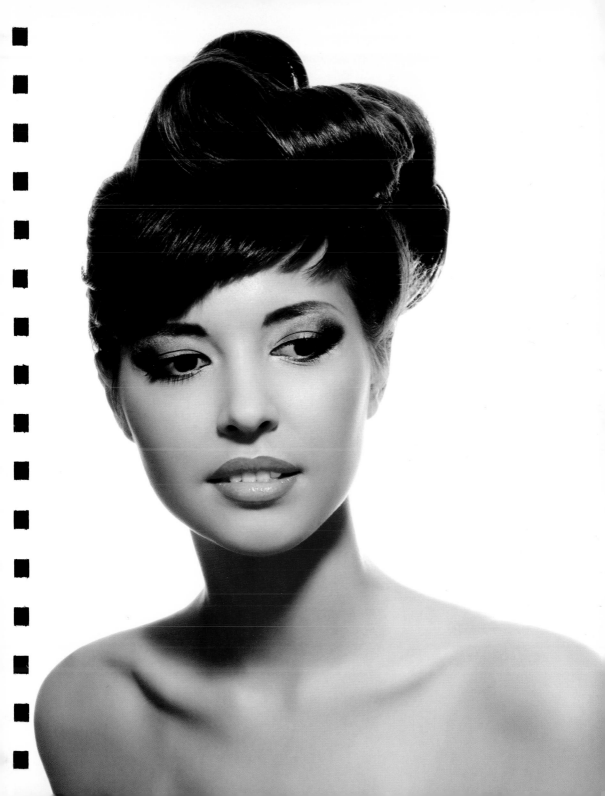

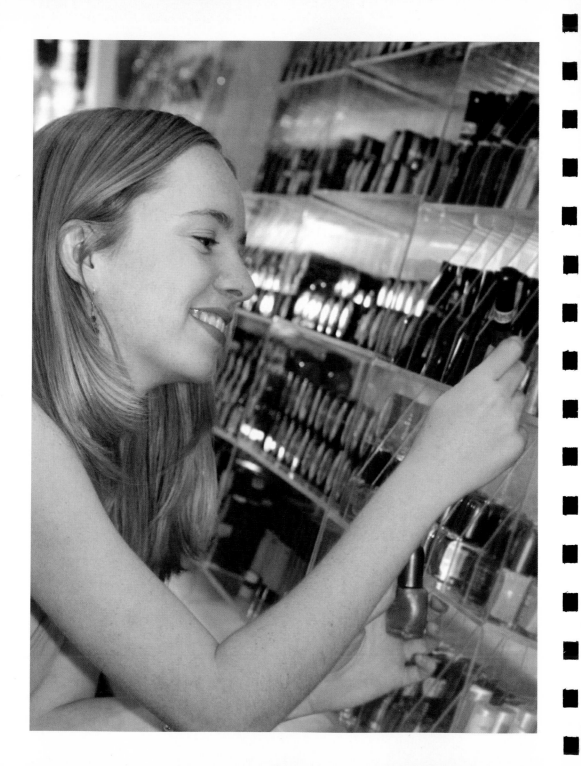

color may be different. The key to success is mastering the basic techniques and becoming competent at a few key makeup looks that work for you.

If you are planning to do your own makeup on your wedding day, in the bridal section (see page 182) you will find looks to suit all skin tones and ages, as well as tips and advice on how to do makeup that will look great from a distance. This is how many of your guests and initially the groom will see you, so your makeup must work in photographs without being too much when the guests and groom are close by.

Also covered in this book are tips and suggested looks for doing makeup on others such as children's face painting and costume parties, and advice on taking makeup further as a career or hobby.

Shopping for makeup

There is an overwhelming amount of makeup available in drugstores, beauty supply shops, and department stores. It can be daunting; so many products to choose from and the pressure to buy can put anyone off. But don't get stuck in a rut and end up using just one brand: be open-minded. A salesperson for a makeup brand may say you need their concealer, foundation, under-eye brightener, and powder for a flawless look, but the tone of the concealer, for example, may not suit your skin, while the concealer from the next counter may be the right match.

The price of makeup products can vary greatly between the brands sold in beauty supply shops and the ones sold at the drugstore. As a general rule you get what you pay for—an eyeshadow or lipstick that costs more money will have more pigment in it, so the color will be stronger and truer to the color on the box when it has been transferred to your skin. The ingredients in an expensive foundation will be better quality and kinder to your skin. On the other hand, I generally would not recommend paying too much for mascara or lip gloss, as they are both highly disposable items and there usually isn't much difference between the formulations available. If you are looking to save money, look for foundations that aren't chalky, concealers that aren't too thin in consistency, and eye and lip pencils that are soft and easily draw a line on the back of your hand without the need to apply too much pressure. Before you go shopping, set a budget and don't spend beyond it. This will stop you from getting coaxed into purchases you have no intention of making. Often, products on beauty counters are not priced, so make sure you ask before you get to the register and get a nasty surprize!

Get to know your makeup. It should all work together—a really strong green eyeshadow is not going to work if you don't have other tones to complement it. The key to makeup shopping is knowing your makeup so well you can spot any gaps. Separate your makeup kit into two bags, drawers, or boxes. The first kit should contain the key products that form the basis of all your makeup looks—this will be your foundation, concealer, powder, bronzer, blush, everyday lip color or gloss, and eye basics. The second bag contains your smoky eye colors and the bright eyeshadow that looks great with your favorite dress or the pink lipstick that makes you feel you can go from day to night in your work suit. When you go shopping, know which kit you are shopping for. Build up the basic kit with quality products rather than quantity. Your second kit is where the frivolous purchases go; this can be as big or as small as you like.

Don't be afraid to ask for application advice and a demonstration from the makeup artist at the counter. Pay attention to what he or she says and if they aren't busy ask if they wouldn't mind watching you apply the product to correct your technique. When I give makeup lessons, I find this is the best way of helping people improve their skills.

Chapter 1

BEFORE YOU GET STARTED

Achieving a professional finish doesn't have to take hours if you look after your skin and know your face and features well. That way you will choose the right product and use it in the right way.

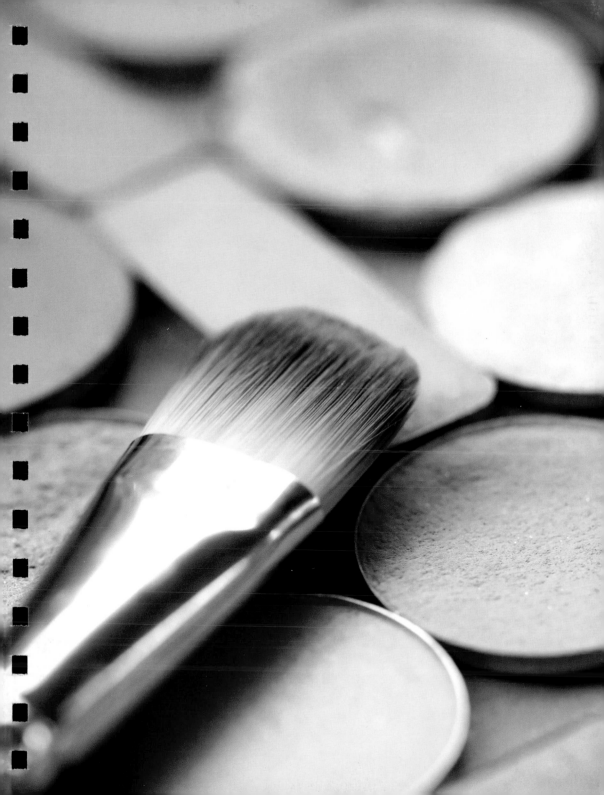

FACE SHAPES

Throughout history, different face shapes have gone in and out of fashion. In the eighteenth century, a widow's peak (one of the characteristics of a heart-shaped face) was the height of fashion, and men wore wigs to re-create this face shape.

There are five main face shapes. By determining what shape your face is, you will be able to get a better understanding of how makeup can work for you. To determine your face shape, stand in front of a mirror and pull your hair back so it is completely off your face; then read the following characteristics of the main face shapes and decide which best describes your face.

KNOWING YOUR FACE

Each face is individual and the features that make up the face are what give it its individuality and beauty. Learning to work with your face shape and features will give you confidence in how you look. The shape of your face is determined by your bone structure; the most flattering face shape is oval. Once you have identified your face shape, you can use contouring and highlighting to alter slightly the shape your face appears to be.

Square face

A square face has a strong, squared jawline, and a broad forehead. Like a round face, the width and length are in proportion, but the main difference between a round face and a square one is that the corners are more angular than curved. The main areas to contour are the temples and outer corners of the jaw, and areas to highlight are the center of the forehead and down the nose. (See page 63.) Blush should be applied vertically on either side of the nose to soften its width.

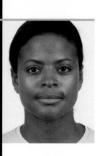
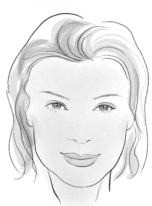

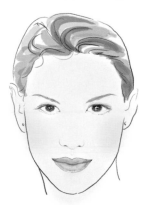
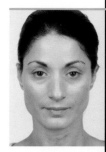

Long face

A long face is longer than it is wide. The forehead, cheekbones, and jawline are typically all the same width. To reduce the length of the face, contour on the chin and along the hairline. Highlight on top of the cheekbone and apply blush horizontally. (See page 64.)

Oval face

The oval face is considered to be the ideal shape because of its balanced proportions. The natural angles are perfect for applying makeup. An oval face has a forehead that is wider than the chin, and prominent cheekbones. An oval face can carry all makeup looks.

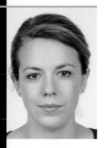

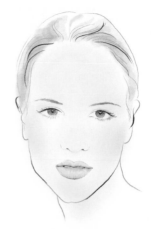

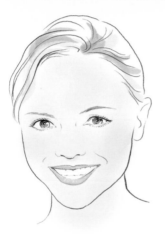

Heart-shaped face

The heart-shaped face is similar to oval, being wide at the forehead, but it then curves down to a point at the chin. The chin can be softened with shading and highlighting, and the forehead can be balanced with shading on the temples. Applying blush on the apples of the cheeks will soften the overall shape. (See page 64.)

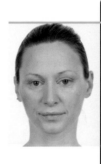

Round face

A round face is youthful looking. The width and length of a round face are in proportion and there are no angles. The cheekbones are hidden by full, wide cheeks. To enhance the appearance of a round face and to bring out the angles and cheekbones, use contouring and highlighting techniques and apply blush on the underside of the cheekbone at a slant. (See page 63.)

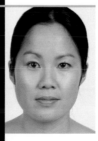

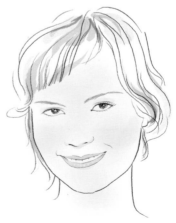

ABOUT EYES

Traditionally, eyes are known as the windows to the soul. They are your most expressive facial feature and your best beauty asset. As well as varying in color, eyes come in many shapes and sizes. By identifiying the specific shape and the setting of your eyes, you can tailor your makeup to enhance them and bring out their natural beauty. The correct eye makeup can totally change your appearance, making small eyes appear bigger or close-set eyes appear wider apart.

Eye care

Eyes are very fragile organs and looking after them is often overlooked. Taking good care of your eyes is absolutely necessary, even when you have no problems. Conjunctivitis is the most common eye problem and is spread very easily. Never use someone else's mascara, and change your own regularly.

Eye makeup should always be thoroughly removed at the end of the day with an eye makeup remover, and a suitable eye cream should be applied around the orbital bone.

If you wear contact lenses, it is very important to wash your hands thoroughly before handling them. When you are putting in your lenses, your eyes should be free of makeup to prevent particles of mascara being trapped underneath them. Never use a cleaning solution that is out-of-date.

- Smoking leads to eyes that are prone to soreness and dehydration.
- It is vital to protect your eyes from UV rays by wearing appropriate glasses or sunglasses when it is bright outside.

Eye makeup for those who wear glasses

- Don't compensate for wearing glasses by piling on loads of eye makeup.
- If you are nearsighted, your eyes can appear smaller behind your glasses, so it is a good idea to line along the top lashes to make them appear bigger. Use a brighter shade of eyeshadow.
- If you are farsighted, the opposite is true; your eyes can appear bigger, so use a darker color over the lid.
- When deciding what kind of eye look to do, consider your frames. If you have heavy frames, go for a more natural look. For light or rimless frames, go more dramatic.
- Glasses draw attention to your brows so make sure they are a good shape and well-groomed.
- To open the eyes and stop your lashes catching against your glasses, curl them before applying mascara.
- Glasses can cast a shadow under the eyes, so use an illuminator to brighten under the eyes.

Eye set and structure

The following illustrations show variations in the set and structure of the eyes, with tips on how to enhance and work with them using makeup.

Close-set eyes

Eyes that are a little too close together, usually narrower than one eye-width, are considered close-set. Making them lighter on the inner corner will widen the appearance of the eyes. To enhance the effect further, extend the outer corners by using darker colors on the outer third of the eye. When you are doing your mascara, always brush the outer lashes out. Apply highlighter just below the outer corners of the lower lashes to draw attention to the outside of the eyelid.

Deep-set eyes

A deep-set eye has a socket that is recessed and the mobile area of lid is small. This creates a lot of natural shadow below the eyes so this area may well need lightening with concealer or highlighter. Light shadow used on the lid with a deep color just above, but not in, the socket line will enhance deep-set eyes and bring them forward. Line both upper and lower lids very close to the lashes.

Wide-set eyes

Eyes are wide-set when the space between the inner corners is wider than the width of one eye. To make the eyes appear closer together, you should use darker shadow in the inner corners, fading to a lighter color on the outer corner. Your eyebrows should not extend beyond the outer corner of the eye and the inner edges should be kept close together. Use eyeliner along the top and bottom lashes. Brush lashes straight up when applying mascara.

Small eyes

Small eyes look proportionately smaller than the rest of the facial features. To enlarge small eyes, apply lighter shades of eyeshadow over the whole eyelid, starting at the lashes, and blending toward the brow. Apply a darker shade of eyeshadow on the outer corner of the eyelid and outer edge of the crease. Use matte white eyeshadow under your brow bone to 'open the eye. Line along the top and bottom lash lines with a soft brown liner, and use a pale pink pencil inside the lower eyelid. Avoid thick black eyeliner, which when ringed completely around the eye makes it appear smaller. Well-shaped brows will make small eyes appear bigger. Curl the eyelashes and apply two coats of mascara to accentuate them.

Round eyes

To elongate round eyes and make them appear more almond-shaped, apply a light-colored eyeshadow on the inner corner of the eye, fading into a medium-colored shadow across the middle of the lid. Next use a dark color on the outer third of the eye and extend it beyond the outer corner, blending downward along the lower lash line. Line along the top and bottom lashes, flicking the line out slightly from the outer corner on the top lid. Build mascara up more on the outer half of the eyelid.

Asian eyes

These eyes have a natural lift at the outer corner. The eyelid is typically small and the crease shallow. Using darker eyeshadow in and above the crease can increase the depth of the eyes. Apply eyeliner as close as possible to the lash line. It can be hard to curl the lashes as they are often quite short, so use individual false eyelashes to enhance the lash line.

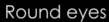

Almond eyes

Almond eyes are well-balanced and considered to have the perfect proportions. This eye shape suits a variety of looks so experiment with different eye makeup and don't hold back! Use eyeliner on the upper lid to make the eyes appear bigger and apply mascara on the upper lashes, emphasising the outer corner. Eyebrows should be groomed to accentuate the eyes. Leave the inner corner of the brow slightly thicker.

Large eyelids

If you have a lot of visible lid from the lashes to the crease, you need to be careful when applying eyeshadow. Keep color close to the lash line, fading out toward the crease across the width of the eyelid. You should not shade in the crease or take color above it. Matte colors work better on large eyelids.

Droopy eyelids

The outer edge of the eyelid tapers downward, which can make you look tired. Lighten under the outer corner of the eye with a pale concealer or a highlighter. Line along the top lash line only and lift the line slightly at the outer corner. Use a neutral shade of eyeshadow over the lid and gradually fade to a darker color above the crease, concentrating on the outer half of the eye.

Hooded eyelids

The eyelid is mostly hidden by a fold of skin from above the socket. Don't avoid eyeshadow on the eyelid, as it will be visible when you blink. With your eye open, make a mark on the upper eye about half a centimeter above the point that your eyelid masks, and take your eyeshadow up to this point so it is visible when your eye is open. Soften the shadow toward the brow so there are no hard lines. Apply a lighter color on the inner corner to open the eye.

ABOUT LIPS

Lips are made of much thinner skin than the skin that covers the rest of your face. Because of this, the blood cells show through, making your lips look red. With darker skin this effect is less prominent because the skin of the lips contains more melanin, making it appear thicker than it is. The lip skin is hairless and has none of its own sweat or sebaceous glands; as a result it lacks the usual protecting layer of sweat and body oils, which keep the skin smooth, inhibit pathogens, and regulate warmth. For these reasons, the lips dry out faster and become chapped more easily—so they need regular moisturizing and even more protection from the sun than the rest of your skin.

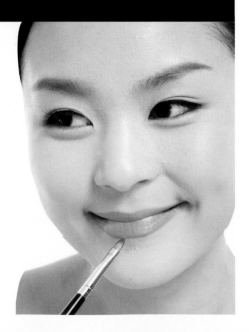

Full lips

- Don't over-line the lips.
- Keep color within the lip line.
- Keep the color soft for day—anything too dark can be overwhelming.
- Matte or gloss colors look good on full lips.

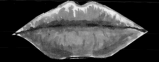

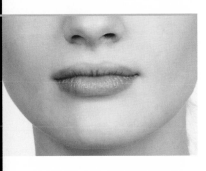

Thin lips

- You can use rich colors as long as you have shaped the lip, and use a touch of shine in the middle.
- Don't use really dark colors.
- Use a liner to even out the shape.
- Apply gloss in the center of the lips to add depth.
- Lip plumpers will increase blood flow and make the lips appear fuller.

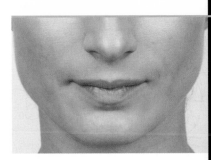

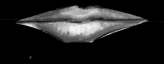

Small bowed lips

- Use a liner to fill out the sides of the top lip slightly and even out the shape.
- Be careful with dark colors.
- Accentuate the natural bow—this is what everyone else is trying to achieve!

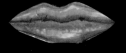

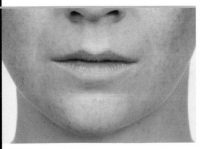

Mature lips

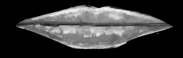

- Use a primer and lipliner to prevent bleeding.
- Some colors will enhance any redness in the face.
- Make lips a focus if you find color on the eyes hard to apply or draining.

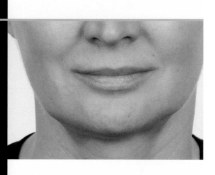

Wide lips

- Use a liner to emphasize the bow in the center of the top lip.
- Matte lipstick can make the lips look very flat, so use gloss to give depth to the lips.
- If you are doing a strong eye look, use a nude on the lips because a stronger color on the lips will be too much.
- Line inside the lip line if you want to play down the lips.

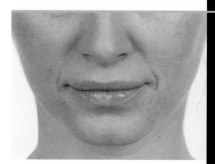

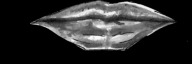

Choosing lip color

- **Dark skin** Plums, wines, and deep reds are flattering for dark skin.
- **Light skin** Light-brown beiges with pink or orange undertones look good on lighter skin.
- **Olive skin** Brownish reds, light browns, and raisin shades suit olive skins.

- **Light colors** For daytime; go darker at night.
- **Sheer and cream** These finishes are more subtle for daytime whereas matte or high-gloss finish add more glamour for night.
- **Shine** A little shine is nice in the day, but matte is professional for the workplace.

SKIN TYPES

The skin consists of three layers: the epidermis on the surface, the dermis, and the subcutaneous fat layer.

Determine your skin type in the morning when the natural oils (or lack of) are most visible to sight and touch. Most people do not have the same texture all over their face, which is what the term "combination skin" refers to. If you do have the same texture all over your skin, it is what is referred to as "normal." Excessive visible surface oil means you have "oily skin," and patchy, flaky skin is known as "dry."

Whatever your skin type, you should use at least an SPF 15 during the day.

Normal skin

Normal skin has an even tone and a smooth texture, with no greasy or flaky areas. Occasionally hormonal breakouts may affect normal skin, but acne is not a problem. It may seem like the lowest maintenance of all skin types but you should not neglect a regular skincare routine as this can lead to signs of aging and wrinkling. It is not uncommon to have normal skin that changes throughout the year from normal to oily, to normal, to dry. You should adapt your routine to suit these changes.

Oily skin

Oily skin has open pores and is prone to blockages that lead to blemishes and blackheads.
A characteristic of oily skin is a shiny T-zone.

The biggest misconception about oily skin is that it should be stripped of all surface oils by using harsh cleansers and toners. This will only cause the skin to produce more oils and in bigger quantities, as it goes into overdrive to try to replenish the lost oils.

Use cleanser in both morning and evening and follow with an alcohol-free toner, such as rosewater. Moisturize all over with a lightweight oil-free moisturizer. An oil-based cleanser that is washed off with warm water actually helps control the surface oiliness. Exfoliate up to three times a week, using a granular exfoliator, and focus on the oiliest areas. Once a week use a clay-based face mask. Use a water-based rather than an oil-based foundation. Don't be tempted by a powder-based foundation as these can go patchy very quickly on oily skin. The advantages of oily skin—yes, there are some!—are that it will show signs of age later and has a strong elasticity, so it will not sag as quickly as other skin types.

Dry skin

Dry skin feels tight, especially after washing with water. Closed pores and no congestion or blackheads are characteristic of dry skin. It can have a tendency for fine wrinkles, flaking, and redness. On darker skin tones dryness can make the skin appear ashy or dull from dead skin buildup. Don't confuse dry skin with dehydrated skin. Dry skin is lacking in oil and dehydrated skin is lacking in moisture.

Remove makeup with a cream or milk cleanser, massaging it into the skin. Rosewater is a gentle toner and doesn't contain alcohol. Use a rich moisturizer in the morning, and at night use night cream or, better still, a night oil. Avoid wetting and drying the skin too often as this promotes dryness.

It is important to exfoliate dry skin once a week as dead skin can build up, making it hard for your moisturizer to penetrate into the skin and also giving it a dull appearance. Use a cream-based exfoliator.

In the morning let your moisturizer settle into your skin and then use a moisturizing foundation. If you have a shiny T-zone dust lightly with translucent powder, but don't use it with a heavy hand and don't apply with a powder puff as the product will collect around any flaky skin. Use a cream blush instead of powder.

Eating oily fish or taking an omega supplement helps oil production and is beneficial to dry skin.

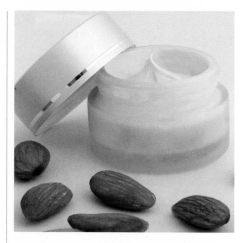

Dehydrated skin

Dry and dehydrated skin are not the same thing. While dry skin is lacking oil, dehydrated skin lacks water content. Dehydration occurs when your skin loses, or is stripped of, more moisture than it is taking in. Moisture in the skin evaporates rapidly and can, therefore, feel tight and itchy, and can appear prematurely aged with fine lines and wrinkles.

Common causes of dehydrated skin are:
- Cleaning the face with soap, which is alkaline and strips the skin of its protective acidic layer.
- Face washes or cleansers, that make your skin feel "squeaky clean."
- Prolonged exposure to air-conditioning or being in a hot, humid climate.
- Neglect: not moisturizing, not drinking enough water, consuming too much alcohol, or smoking.
- Using astringent face wipes that contain alcohol will strip the skin of natural oils.

To combat dehydrated skin drink lots of water, use an oil-based cleanser, and avoid products that contain alcohol such as makeup wipes. Always use moisturizer in the morning and at night use a heavier night cream or a combination of moisturizer and serum.

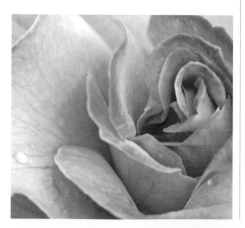

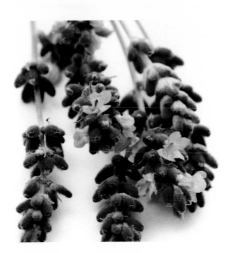

Combination skin

Combination skin can be a combination of any of the other skin types. It can be both oily and dry, or dry and sensitive. It is very common to be oily in the middle of the face, on the nose, forehead, and chin, but have some dryness on the cheeks or around the mouth or eyes. You should treat the prevailing type of skin. Look for cleansing products that are suitable for combination skin as it is quite hard and time-consuming to isolate the separate areas of your face when removing your makeup. If there are areas of dryness, they should be treated with a heavier moisturizer than areas of oiliness.

If you have an oily T-zone, use a light powder to control shine, but avoid using powder on the dry areas. Use a cream blush instead of a powder one if you have any dryness on your cheeks.

Sensitive skin

Sensitive skin tends to be thin, with broken capillaries. It reacts quickly to both heat and cold so is prone to redness and flushes. It is commonly dry and frequently suffers from allergic reactions. Temperature changes, detergents, makeup, fragrance, and alcohol in skincare products can all cause irritation, leaving the skin red and blotchy.

Always patch-test products by applying a small amount behind your ear. Over the next 24 hours, montior the area to see if any redness or irritation has occurred.

You should use skincare that is mild and does not contain potential allergens. Use cream or milk cleansers, which contain calming ingredients such as lavender. Avoid hot water; instead use lukewarm water on your face. When your face is wet pat dry instead of rubbing. Choose a moisturizer that is designed for sensitive skin and stick to ones with few ingredients. Exfoliate with a gentle cream exfoliator, not a granular one.

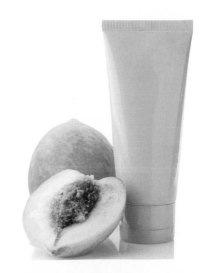

SKIN TONES

The color of skin can range from nearly colorless to almost black. The color of an individual's skin is determined by the amount and type of melanin in the skin. Melanin is the pigment that gives color to the hair, skin, and eyes and helps protect the skin from the sun. The variation in skincolor can mainly be put down to genetics. People whose ancestors come from warmer tropical regions have darker skin than people from cooler climates.

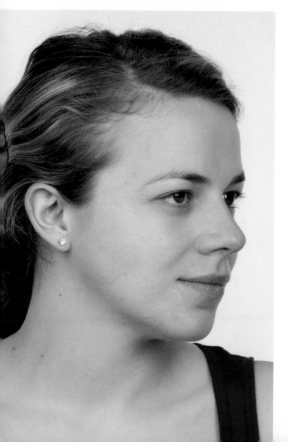

Regardless of skin tone, all women are striving to make their skin appear smooth and flawless. To do this you need to follow a good skincare regime and choose the correct shade of foundation and concealer to work with the tones of your skin. You also need to acknowledge that your skin condition and color can vary with the seasons.

⊕ Fair skin

White skin, which is pale but more creamy than translucent. This skin tone is very easy to work with; it suits most colors of blush, lip, and eye makeup. Variations in hair color can affect color choice for lips and eyes. The foundation should match the skin tone, and warmth can be added with bronzer. The overall look should still be subtle, so build up the color slowly.

⊕ Pale skin

The fairest skins have very little color and can appear almost translucent. Extra care must be taken in the sun, as this skin burns very easily. Makeup should be transparent and delicate for a barely-there effect. Use a sheer base and add cover with concealer where required. I would always advise using a foundation that matches your skincolor, as using a darker shade of foundation than your skin looks very unnatural. Choose a subtle blush color—anything with too much pigment can make you look like a clown. Soft pinks or apricot work well, and avoid anything with a brown undertone. If your eyebrows are very fair, darken them slightly with brow powder to add definition. Pale lashes need mascara; for a more natural look use brown. Don't go for heavy makeup looks during the day because they can look harsh. Cool subtle tones are the way to go.

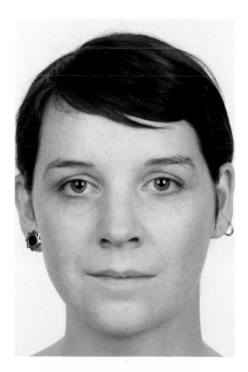

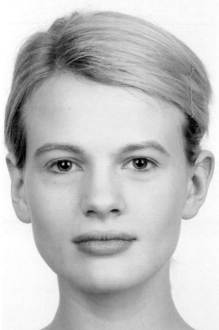

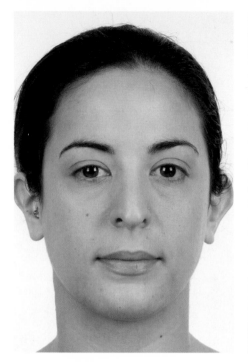

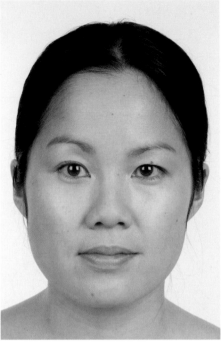

⊕ Caramel

Asian women should use a caramel-colored foundation with yellow undertones. These will enhance the natural color of the Asian skin tone. Choosing foundation that has pink undertones will result in skin that looks either too orange, or chalky and ghostlike. Asian skin can sometimes look sallow, so warm it up with bronzer on the high points of the face. A common problem is darkness under the eyes, so you may need to layer concealer, starting with a pink- or peach-toned corrector and finishing with a concealer with yellow undertones that matches the color of the skin. Women with an Asian skin tone are complemented by soft warm colors and smoky kohl-lined eyes. Avoid eye makeup that is paler than the skin tone.

⊕ Warm almond

Many women with a warm almond skin tone believe they should use foundation with a pink undertone. Matching foundation to skin tone always gives the most natural look, so choose a foundation with a yellow undertone. Asian women are susceptible to sunspots and sun damage, so they should always wear sunscreen. Don't be tempted to use a heavy foundation all over the face; use a normal weight foundation and use peachy-toned concealer for additional cover where required. Rich colors look great on Asian eyes.

◑ Olive

An olive tone is characterized by a golden complexion. The skin tans easily but can have a yellow/green undertone in winter, because although it appears yellow it has a natural green undertone as well as yellow. Use bronzer to warm the skin during this time. A couple of foundations will be required to match to the skincolor because it varies throughout the year. Choose two colors in the darkest and lightest colors of your skin; you can then mix them in varying quantities to achieve anything in-between. Choose blushes in shades such as warm pink, coral, apricot, terracotta, dark plum, and bronze. These will provide a natural glow. Avoid colors that are too bright or too pale.

◑ Dark

There are many different tones of black skin. In general black skin tends to be lighter in the middle of the face and darker across the forehead and around the perimeter. Foundation should be used to even out the different tones seamlessly, which may mean you need a couple of different shades. Whichever tones you decide to play up, always choose foundation with warm, rich undertones to avoid looking too chalky or ashy. Dark skin does not normally require a heavy foundation because redness, sunspots, and blemishes are not as visible as on paler skins; in most instances, a tinted moisturizer offers enough cover. Concealer can give additional cover where needed. Blush enhances the skin tone and features. A deeper pigment is required than on paler skins. Women with dark skin can use color on their eyes to very dramatic effect.

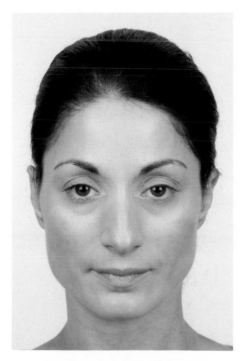

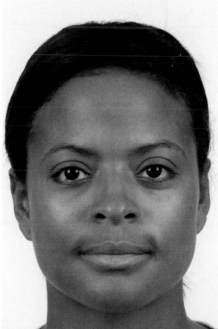

SKIN PREPARATION

Your skin should be smooth and well moisturized.
A good diet, drinking lots of water, and a regular skincare
routine using the correct products for your skin type and
age, will lead to glowing skin that remains youthful for as
long as possible. Good skin is something that you need to
work at constantly, and there is no quick fix. Before
applying your makeup, preparing your skin correctly will
reduce irritation, protect your skin, and extend the
wearing time of your makeup.

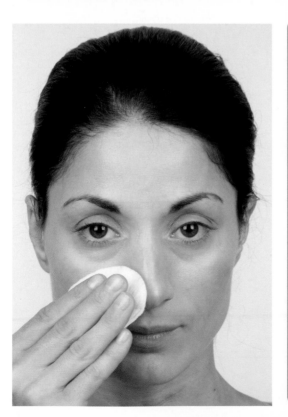

Dangers of soap

You shouldn't use normal soap on
your face that you would use to
wash your body. The skin on your
face is thin and easily irritated, so
it needs a more gentle cleanser.
Soap dries the skin, stripping it of
the natural oils that are needed to
protect it against environmental
damage. The oils also stop pores
from getting clogged with airborne
dust and dirt. Even if you have
oily skin and think it helps prevent
breakouts and acne, you should
switch to a cleanser, face wash, or
face soap specifically formulated
for your skin type. Normal soap may
achieve short-term results for oily
skin, but you should have a longer-
term approach to skin care.

Exfoliator

Depending on your skin type, you should exfoliate 1–3 times a week. Exfoliating removes dead skin cells from the surface of the skin, giving it a radiant, natural glow.

Exfoliating also allows your skincare products to work better as they can penetrate through the top layers of the skin with more ease.

Always exfoliate the skin when it is clean, and don't use exfoliator to remove makeup.

There are different types of exfoliator, which are suitable for different skin types:

Chemical Freshens the skin by gently dissolving the dead skin on the surface. It is left on the skin for 5–10 minutes and then washed away. Less abrasive than a granular exfoliator.

Cream A very gentle exfoliator, which is good for sensitive skin. It is applied in a thin layer and left to dry completely, then rubbed off. This dissolves the dead skin, which rubs away with the exfoliator.

Granular A more abrasive exfoliator which polishes the skin as well as removing the dead cells and boosting circulation. Good for oily or combination skin, the exfoliator is massaged into the skin and then removed with a muslin facial cloth, or by splashing with water. The benefits are increased if you use it in a steamy room or in the shower.

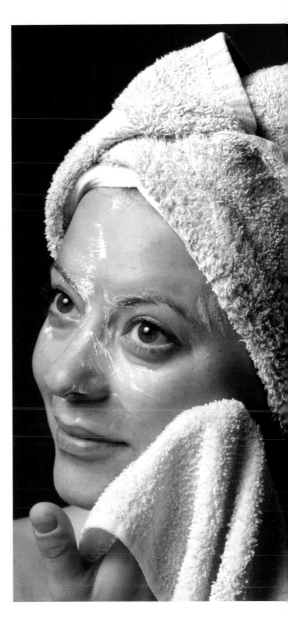

YOUR DAILY ROUTINE

Every day you need to cleanse, hydrate, and protect your skin. Your routine will not be the same in the morning as in the evening and you should factor in a weekly exfoliation. It is really important not to strip the skin of the oils it needs to keep irritants out and moisture in; so do not over-cleanse or use products that are too harsh. The skin on the face is thinner than that on the rest of the body, so it can become sensitive. Oils protect the skin against environmental damage caused by changes in temperature, wind, and rain. The most damaging environmental factor is the sun; even on a cloudy day its rays can cause damage. If you like a tanned look, use fake tan products and always wear at least an SPF 15.

In the morning

Your skin needs a wake-up. Depending on its type this might just mean splashing it with cold water, or if your skin is oily you can use a gentle face wash. This should be followed with a lightweight daytime moisturizing cream or lotion, ideally with an SPF. You should also use eye cream around the delicate eye area.

In the evening

It is important to clean your face to remove your makeup and the impurities that collect on the surface during the day. You should do this with a proper cream or wash cleanser, not wipes or soap. To remove eye makeup—especially mascara—you should use an eye makeup remover. Normal cleansers can contain fragrance or ingredients that are not suitable to use on the delicate area around the eyes. You should then apply eye cream and a night moisturizer or serum, or both. The combination of products will depend on your skin type and age.

Your skin renews itself at night while you are sleeping, so specific night products contain ingredients to aid this process.

Weekly

Exfoliate at least once a week. This removes dead skin cells and improves the texture of the surface of the skin, as well as aiding circulation and keeping the layers under the surface plumped.

Face masks also improve the health and appearance of the skin. There are many different masks available that treat different problems or encourage radiance and vitality. For example, you can use a clay-based one to control oiliness, or a cream one for hydration. Steam is also excellent for clearing congestion.

Your skin will also benefit from professional treatments such as facials. There are many different types available. Sometimes a course of treatments is recommended rather than just one pick-me-up. Take advice from your local beauty salon.

Basic preparation

➔ step 1

In the morning your skin is clean from the night before, so splash with water to freshen and close pores. If surface oiliness is a problem, soak a cotton pad in toner and wipe over either the whole face or just the T-zone. Moisturize with daytime cream or lotion.

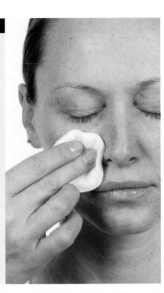

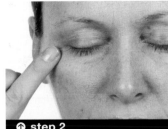

⬆ step 2

Apply eye cream. Instead of dragging it or rubbing into the skin, tap it on, working all the way around the orbital bone (eye socket). Rubbing encourages the skin to sag, and tapping increases the blood circulation and plumps the surface of the skin.

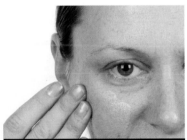

⬆ step 3

When you are ready to apply your makeup, start by applying primer. There are different primer formulations available (see page 42), for example a primer with a green tint, as used here, will counteract redness. You may find you don't need both moisturizer and primer. They don't do the same job, but your skin may not be able to absorb both simultaneously.

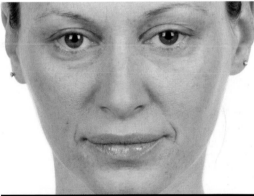

⬆ step 4

Good skin preparation will lead to a better makeup application, which is easier to do, lasts longer, and has a more professional finish.

Chapter 2

ESSENTIAL TECHNIQUES

The saying "don't run before you can walk" is very relevant when it comes to makeup application. Most of us probably can't remember when we first wore makeup and we certainly wouldn't have been taught how to apply it. So our makeup routines have developed from crude beginnings of trial and error and imitating pictures in magazines.

This chapter takes you through the basics. Take time to go back to the beginning, forget your old methods of applying makeup, and learn how to apply it the professional way.

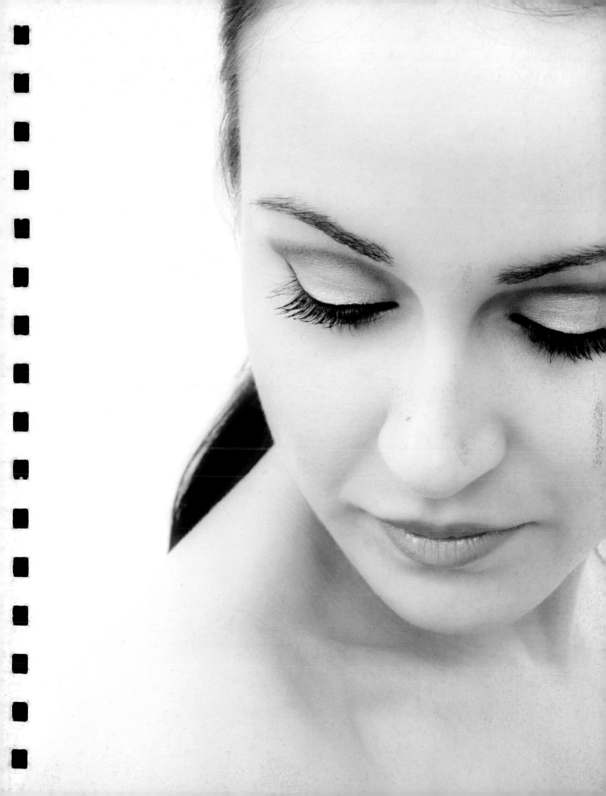

EQUIPMENT

If you have a good range of high-quality makeup products, you need to have good tools with which to apply them. Otherwise the money you have spent on products will have been wasted. You can buy makeup brushes from professional shops that carry their own line, as well as at many department store makeup counters.

It is definitely worth splashing out on good-quality powder, blush, and eyeshadow brushes; those made from real animal hair are the best. You can buy them at department store beauty counters or from professional suppliers (see page 248). Don't buy store-brand or budget powder brushes, because the application will be poor and the bristles will shed quickly. It is easy to tell a good-quality brush by testing the bristles on your hand; it will feel scratchy if it is poor quality and synthetic hair.

For applying foundation and cream products such as concealer, cake eyeliner, and lipstick, brushes made from synthetic hair and sold in drugstores will be fine.

For powder, blush, and contouring

Powder brush The dome shape is to ensure that powder gets an even application on the whole face, around the edges of the nose, and under the eyes. It should be made of real hair and feel soft and fluffy to the touch.

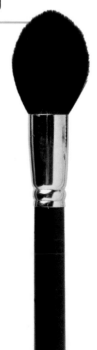

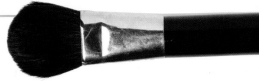

Blush brush The bristles should be real hair and feel soft. The edges of the brush are rounded for natural application. The brush should feel firmer than the powder brush against the back of your hand.

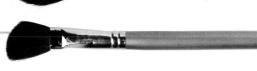

Contouring brush This brush should be made of real hair and feel soft but firm. It has a tapered head, which enables you to apply contouring blush in the correct place by turning the brush so that the longer hairs are closer to the jawline and the shorter hairs are closer to the cheekbone.

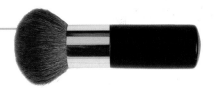

Bronzer brush This brush is made of real hair that is very densely packed, with a stout but rounded head. It is used to push bronzer into the cheeks and highpoints of the face for a natural-looking finish.

For foundation and concealer

Foundation brush This brush is made of synthetic fibers and has a flat edge. It ensures the foundation is applied evenly and gets into all corners.

Concealer brush Made from synthetic fibers with a rounded head, it is much smaller than the foundation brush and used for applying concealer around the eyes, as well as for detail work in creases, on blemishes, or around the edges of the nose and lips.

Fiber-optic foundation brush This brush is relatively new and is excellent for blending over the face after you have applied your foundation, and for buffing foundation to an airbrush finish that will look flawless. Don't use this brush to apply foundation directly to the face, as the bristles soak up too much product.

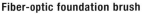

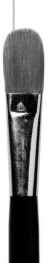

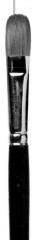

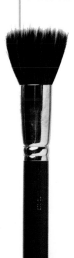

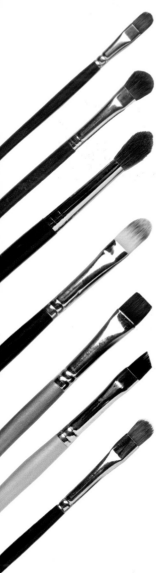

For eyes

Medium-head eyeshadow brush This brush should be made of real hair that is densly packed so feels firm. It is flat with a rounded edge so that it can easily blend eyeshadow over the rounded shape of the eye.

Large-head eyeshadow brush The same as the medium brush but used for covering a larger area. Ideal for the application of base eyeshadow colors or a wash of color.

Eyeshadow blending brush This is made of real hair and has a dome-shaped head with longer bristles than the other eyeshadow brushes. It should be soft and fluffy to touch and is used for blending eyeshadows together and softening edges. It can also be used for applying powder under the eyes to set concealer.

Cream eyeshadow brush Used for the application of cream eyeshadow products, this brush is flat with a rounded head, similar to the medium eyeshadow brush, but is made of synthetic fibers. It can also be used to touch up foundation and concealer.

Flat liner brush Made of synthetic bristles and flat with a square edge, this brush is used for precision and easy application of cake or gel eyeliner close to the lash line.

Slanted eyebrow brush Made of synthetic bristles that are flat with a slanted edge. This brush is used to fill and enhance the eyebrows with eyebrow powder.

Eye detail brush This brush is the same shape as the medium and large eyeshadow brushes and is made of real hair but is much smaller and has many uses. It can be used to smudge powder eyeshadow into eyeliner, apply loose pigments with precision, or apply eyeshadow under the bottom lashes close to the root of the lashes.

Using your fingers

I am a big fan of using fingers to blend foundation and concealer. The warmth of the fingers works with the product to blend it into the skin for a natural finish. I would recommend first applying with a foundation brush for a light, even cover, and then using your fingers to blend the product in.

Cleaning your brushes

I recommend cleaning your powder, blush, foundation, and concealer brushes every week to eliminate product buildup and keep bacteria at bay. If you are using similar colors, you should also wash your eyeshadow brushes once a week, but if you do a smoky eye look one day and want to go back to a natural look the next day, you will need to wash the brushes in-between.

You can buy alcohol-based brush cleaners from professional suppliers that are fast-drying and good at dissolving the buildup of cream products on synthetic brushes. Alternatively, use shampoo and warm water. Immerse just the heads of the brushes in the water, otherwise the glue holding the head to the handle will start to break down and the brush will eventually come apart. Rinse the soap out of the brush and blot the excess water out with a towel. Leave the brushes to dry overnight.

Other brushes and tools

1 Lip brush This brush is made of synthetic hair, is flat, and comes to a slight point in the middle. It is used to apply lip color or gloss and to blend lipliner and color together.

2 Lash wand Similar to the wand in a mascara tube, this is used to groom eyebrow hairs into place and to brush through mascara before it dries, if it looks clumpy.

3 Tweezers The difference between a good pair of tweezers and a bad pair is a lot of pain when tidying eyebrows! It pays to invest in a good pair and they will last.

4 Eyelash curlers These are essential and make a huge difference to the appearance of eyelashes. They should always be used before applying mascara, or it will clump. Lightly press the curlers together to ensure you haven't caught any skin and then increase the pressure and hold for 5–10 seconds.

5 Sponges Some people prefer to use a sponge to apply their foundation. I would recommend the disposable wedge-shaped ones. They reach into all the creases and corners for an even application. Because they are designed to be thrown away after one use, there is no product buildup to worry about.

6 Powder puff Used to press powder into the skin for a lasting finish and shine control. A puff should be velour and should be washed regularly. I would recommend having a few.

7 Cotton swabs Widely available in drugstores and supermarkets, disposable cotton swabs are used to smudge eyeliner and clean up any fallen product.

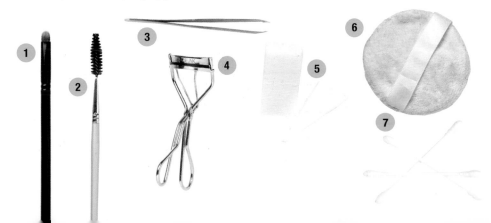

PRODUCTS

Whether you are a makeup junkie or have a strict bare-essentials-only makeup policy, you should have a good-quality basic makeup kit. Refer to page 11 for advice on choosing and shopping for your makeup.

Primer

Using a makeup primer is the best way to get your makeup to last. Makeup primers are relatively new products, but they are gaining in popularity. The aim of a primer is to prepare the skin for makeup application. They pamper the skin and create a protective base for longer-lasting, more natural-looking foundation application and wear. Primers give the makeup something to grab onto and help your makeup last longer, because they create a smooth and perfect surface. They work especially well for people with oily and combination skin because they control excess shine and absorb oil. A makeup primer is also appropriate for those with very dry and sensitive skin, because it nourishes the skin and calms inflammation. Most primers are colorless, but tinted ones are available to treat specific problems such as redness and sallowness.

Benefits of using makeup primers

- Smoother skin surface so smoother finish.
- Even skin tone.
- Disguise skin flaws and imperfections.
- Pamper and nourish.
- Create a protective base for longer-lasting foundation.
- Reduce redness and inflammation.
- Moisturize your skin and keep it hydrated all day long.
- Reduce excess shine on the forehead, nose, and chin.
- Fill in fine lines and wrinkles.
- Make enlarged pores appear smaller and less visible.
- Prevent cosmetics from clogging pores.

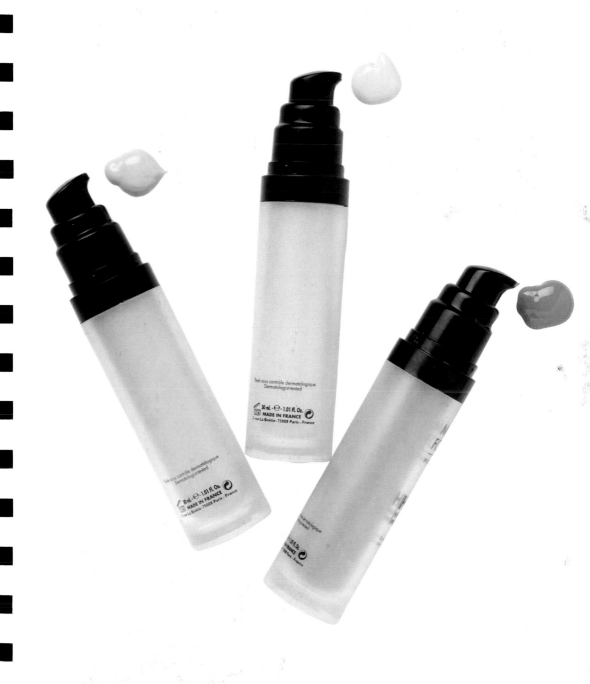

FOUNDATION

The correct formula and shade will give you an even complexion with a healthy glow. A foundation is not just a foundation anymore—modern formulas can double as sunscreen, anti-aging products, and problem treatment creams. It is the most important product in your kit; it is the base over which all other makeup is applied. Don't scrimp when it comes to buying a foundation. Take time to discover your skin type and tone (see pages 25–31) and learn about the different formulations available so you make the right choice for your skin.

Powder Not to be confused with translucent or tinted blotting powder that is used to set makeup and control shine. Good for oily skin and has the quickest application.

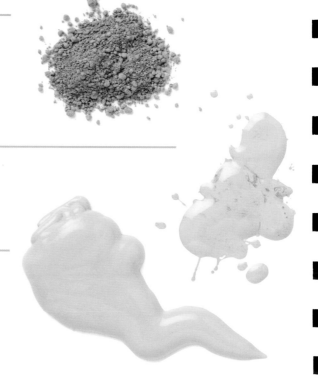

Liquid Easy to blend and achieve an even finish with. It comes in many formulas: normal, dry, sensitive, and oil-free so suits most people. Can be oil- or water-based and gives a medium or heavy coverage.

Tinted moisturizer The lightest foundation, great on clear skin to even out tone, or in the summer when you want a sheer cover. Oil-free is available for oily skins, or try tinted balm for dry skin. You can mix moisturizer into your normal foundation to make it a lighter consistency.

Cream Perfect for older or drier skin, where other formulations may sit on the surface of the skin and be visible.

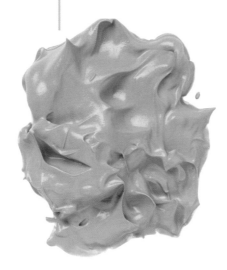

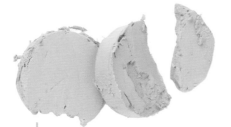

Stick Similar to a cream foundation but with slightly heavier coverage, can be used as both concealer and foundation. The packaging makes it convenient to carry out and about, and application is quick and easy. A good choice for normal to oily skin.

Other blends

Mousse A lightweight whipped foundation; due to the consistency you have more control when you are applying it than with a liquid foundation. It dries quickly so some practice is required. This type of foundation will give a matte finish.

Spray A flawless airbrush finish, hardest to apply—takes some practice. If applied correctly it will have a smooth, velvety finish that you can't necessarily get when applying foundation.

Spray foundation Liquid foundation with air whipped in. It takes some practice to get the application correct, but it can give a smooth, flawless, airbrushed finish that has a great coverage while feeling light.

Mineral powders The latest thing in makeup. They have very few ingredients and, being inert minerals, they tend to be perfect for people who suffer from allergic reactions to makeup, or who have sensitive skin. Apply using a brush and buff into the skin. The coverage and finish of mineral powders does not suit everyone.

Cream to powder Goes on as cream, but dries to a powder finish. It is good for oily skin as it reduces shine, but can look cakey if applied too heavily or if layered on throughout the day. Convenient to carry because it comes in a compact.

COLOR SELECTION

The right tone and formula for you will be invisible when your foundation is applied correctly—you should look like you aren't wearing any!

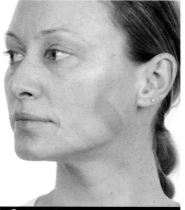

⬆ step 1

Test the color of foundation on the jawline—it should disappear into the skin and blend seamlessly between the face and neck.

➔ step 2

Apply foundation to the face, starting in the center and blending over the nose, working outward over the cheeks, chin, and forehead. Apply with a foundation brush or your fingers.

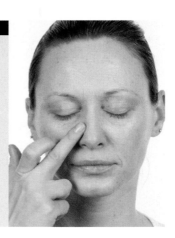

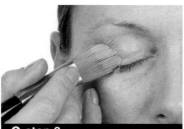

⬆ step 3

The skin of the eyelids is thin, making redness and veins visible. Cover them with a thin layer of foundation; this will act as a base for eye makeup.

➔ step 4

Circle the whole face with a fiber-optic brush for a seamless finish. Make small circles with the brush and cover the whole face from hairline to jaw.

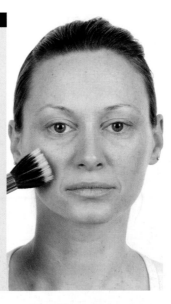

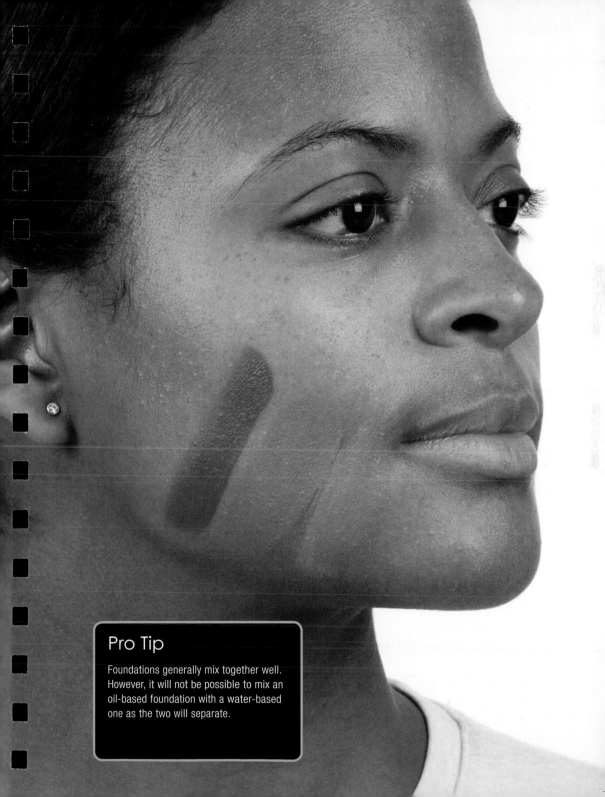

Pro Tip

Foundations generally mix together well.
However, it will not be possible to mix an
oil-based foundation with a water-based
one as the two will separate.

CONCEALER

The purpose of concealer is to cover blemishes, dark circles, redness, broken capillaries, and any other small imperfections of the skin. Heavy camouflage concealer can also be used to cover scars and birthmarks. It is much better to use a lighter formula of foundation and to add more coverage with concealer where required rather than covering the whole face with a heavy foundation. Concealer looks most natural when it has been applied in sheer layers, building up the cover gradually. Ideally you should have two different shades of concealer: one that is one or two shades lighter than your skin tone and one that is one shade darker. These can be blended together to match your skin tone or used alone. Between them they will enable you to flatten a raised blemish, cover all imperfections, and blend areas of discoloration or dark circles under the eyes.

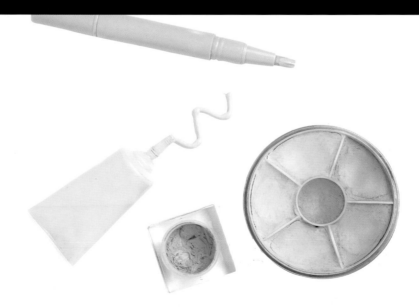

Concealer should have a yellow undertone, the shade of which will depend on your skin tone:

Skin tone	Concealer
very pale	ivory
pale	light beige
almond	light peach
olive	warm beige
caramel	honey
dark	peach/caramel
very dark	cocoa

Avoid concealers that look too pink or white. Using a concealer that is too light under the eye will emphasize the dark area instead of concealing it and will give you panda eyes. The best concealers have a totally smooth texture and are enriched with vitamins.

There are many different formulas of concealer available that provide varying levels of cover and are suitable for use on different areas of the face. The choice of a concealer type depends on your skin type and the area you want to conceal:

Cream Gives full coverage, is creamy and easy to blend so can be used under eyes, and is heavy enough to cover dark circles. Can be in a tube, compact, or pot. The creamiest versions are good for older skin as they are hydrating and are easy to apply without dragging the skin.

Highlighting pens Used on the inner corner of the eye to brighten dark circles and shadows. Can be used in wrinkles to make them appear shallower, around the edges of the mouth, and under the outer corner of the eye to lift.

Color correctors Used to cover discoloration. Use green to counteract redness, lilac for sallowness, yellow for purple or blue-tinged circles. Blue tones down orange, and orange-toned correctors are used to cover a bruise or tattoo.

Camouflage The heaviest concealer, it can be used to cover birthmarks, sunspots, scars, and even tattoos.

Solid stick Perfect for blemishes, provides direct on-the-spot application. The consistency is thick but fairly dry, so it is not so easy to use under the eyes.

Mineral powder Easy application, good for sensitive skin and eyes. Gives light to medium coverage for dark circles and blemishes.

Liquid Usually comes in a wand or pen and gives the lightest coverage. Has a creamy formula and is easy to blend. Multiuse; covers minor blemishes and slight shadows and is good for touch-ups.

Pencils For medium coverage and to use on small imperfections; not suited for shadows and dark circles. Very portable and good for touch-ups.

Pro Tip

Always apply foundation before concealer, otherwise you will move it away when you apply your foundation. This also allows you to see what cover is provided by your foundation and how much additional cover is required from a concealer.

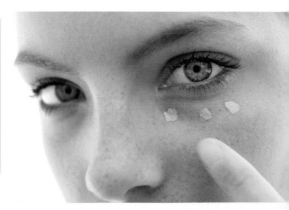

Concealing

It is important to use the correct technique when applying concealer; otherwise, it will be visible and will highlight what you are trying to conceal. The skin under the eye is thinner than elsewhere on the face. On pale skin it can appear transparent and show off the veins that are close to the surface.

➔ step 1

Use a cream or liquid concealer one or two shades lighter than the skin tone to cover dark circles. Apply the product from the inner corner of the eye along the orbital bone approximately a third of the way across the width of the socket. For a precise application, apply with a concealer brush.

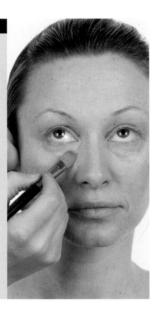

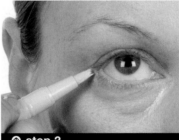

⬆ step 2

Apply eye-brightener on the inner bridge of the nose around the corner of the eye. If there is a visible crease or fold of skin, apply in the crease under the eye to lift and flatten. Also apply under the outer corner of the eye for instant lift.

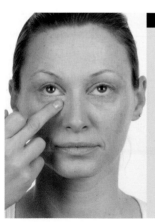

⬅ step 3

Use the pad of your middle finger to tap the concealer into the skin. Tap and lightly rub outward and back inward; don't drag or pull the skin.

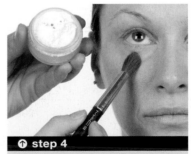

⬆ step 4

Use a yellow-toned powder over the whole eye area to set the concealer and prevent creasing. Use a small dome brush (an eyeshadow blending brush) for precise application.

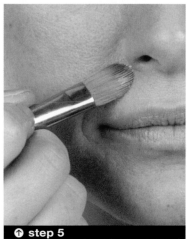

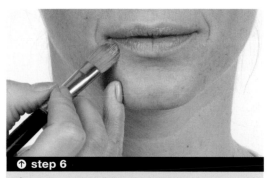

↑ step 6

Conceal around the lipline to enhance the lip shape and stop lipstick from bleeding. Using your eye-brightener under the outer two-thirds of the lower lips will lift the whole lip.

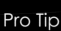 **↑ step 5**

Conceal any redness around the edge of the nose using a fine-tipped concealer brush. This enables you to get right into the corners.

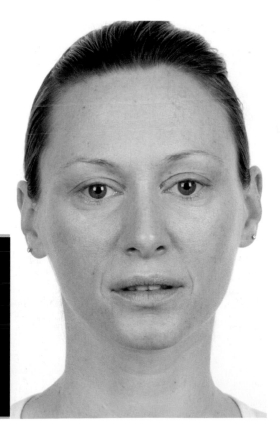

Pro Tip

Concealer is used to lighten around the eyes, whereas on the rest of the face it is used to hide blemishes and imperfections so that they blend with the skin tone. If you use the same product to do both, blemishes can end up being highlighted rather than concealed.

Concealing puffy lower eyelids

Use concealer to reduce the size of a raised lower eyelid, which can look like an eye bag and give a tired appearance.

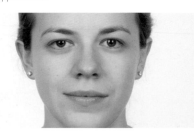

Step 1 To flatten a protruding eyelid, shade with a slightly darker shade of concealer directly on the raised area, from the inner to the outer corner of the eye. Highlight below the raised area, smudging the two shades together so there are no hard edges.
Step 2 Set with a yellow-toned loose powder unless you are very fair, in which case use a white translucent powder.

Pro Tip

Use an eye cream before applying concealer.

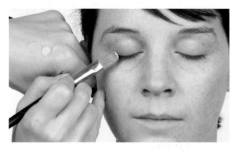

Concealing redness around eyes

Some eyes may need additional cover to create an even base. Neutralize the redness by applying a green primer to the whole area. Conceal under the eye right up to the lash line from corner to corner, then apply the same concealer over the whole eyelid that you use under your eye. Set with loose powder.

Pro Tip

Hyperpigmentation is where the lower layers of the skin have been damaged and have deepened or lightened in color as a result. These areas can be concealed. This should be done before and again after applying foundation if further cover is required.

Concealing dark circles around the eyes

Due to the tone, redness is not such an issue with dark skin as it is with paler skins. Blemishes are also less visible and less common. However, dark circles and hyperpigmentation can be a problem. The primary cause of a predisposition to dark circles is that they are inherited. Although this is not the only cause; sun exposure boosts melanin so can emphasize darkness. Fatigue and illness make skin paler so dark circles appear darker and as we age our skin becomes thinner, so veins are more visible.

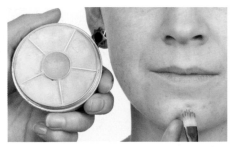

Concealing blemishes

Use a concealer that matches your skin tone (nothing too creamy) over the raised area, using a concealer brush, starting at the center and blending outward until it disappears into the surrounding skin. If it still appears raised, apply a concealer one shade darker than your skin tone onto the raised area. For precise application, use a small concealer brush and gently pat with the pad of your index finger to blend. With a velour puff, press loose powder over the top to set. Press it onto the skin lightly and remove, without disturbing the product.

Concealing dark circles around the eyes

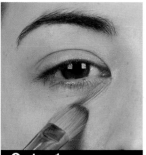

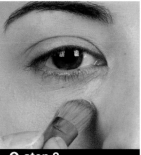

↑ step 1

Apply a peachy-toned corrector to the area under the eye to cover dark circles. Make sure the product covers the inner corner of each eye, as this casts a shadow over the area under the eye.

↑ step 2

Thinly layer on top of this a pink-based corrector, in order to brighten the eye. Smudge a little of this product on the outer corner of the eye to lift it.

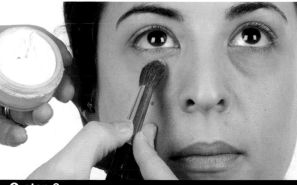

↑ step 3

Set with a yellow-based, loose powder using a small dome (eyeshadow blending) brush. If necessary, add concealer in your normal shade over the top to blend into the rest of the face.

Pro Tips

- Use a peach-toned concealer on dark circles.
- Applying eye-brightener in a crease lifts it to the surface and smooths the appearance of the skin.
- Smudging brightener on the outer corner of the eye with your finger lifts the eyelid.
- Use a yellow-toned powder over the whole eye area to set eye makeup. Apply this with a small dome brush.
- Conceal around the nose using a pink-toned concealer, applied with a synthetic concealer brush.
- Conceal around the lip line to enhance the lip shape using a concealer one shade lighter than the skin tone.

POWDER

The purpose of powder is to maximize the longevity of your makeup by setting the foundation and concealer and controlling shine, especially on the nose, chin, and forehead. Powder should not alter the color of your foundation, so choose a translucent powder or a shade similar to that of your foundation. The darker your skin, the more pigment you will require in the powder. Loose powder is one of the most useful products in your makeup bag. It is used to set foundation and concealer, to protect your face makeup when doing a heavy eye look by piling it on your cheekbones to catch loose product, and to blend the edges of your blush for a really flawless finish. Pressed powder is convenient and portable. It gives a lighter finish than loose powder, which is denser.

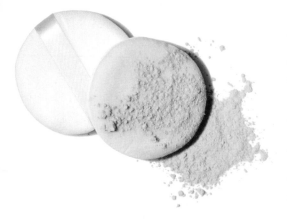

For a matte finish, press powder into the face with a puff and then brush over with a powder brush to remove excess. For a sheerer application, apply with a powder brush, lightly pressing into the skin and then sweeping the brush over. With a smaller dome-shaped brush, apply powder to harder-to-reach areas such as the inner corners and under the eyes, and around the bottom of the nose.

There are some situations where powder or the repeated application of powder is not suitable. If your skin is really dry or flaky, use powder only to set under-eye concealer and lightly counteract shine on the T-zone. Don't use it anywhere else, as it will only emphasize the dryness. If you have oily skin, repeated application of powder can turn your makeup cakey. Use oil-blotting powders as an alternative.

Translucent powder

Is either white or tinted to match skin tone. It is used to set makeup and control shine without adding any color.

Pigmented powder

Toned to match foundation shades. Can be used to set makeup and control shine but don't be too heavy-handed or it can make your foundation look cakey. Sometimes it can darken your foundation, so go for one shade lighter.

Powder foundation

Made to be used as a foundation and powder in one; it is much denser than setting powder. For a sheerer finish, apply with a wet sponge.

Mineral powder

For sensitive skin, has very few ingredients. It has a dewy finish and is used as a foundation.

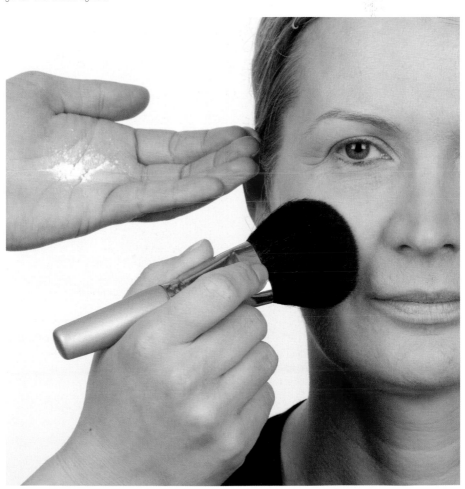

Powder application

Whichever method of application you choose, it is important you keep your tools clean to prevent product buildup, the spread of bacteria, and an uneven finish.

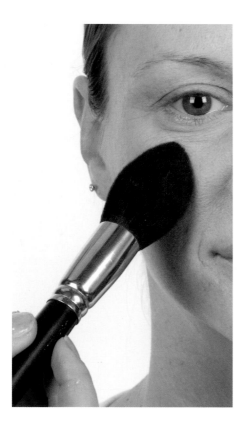

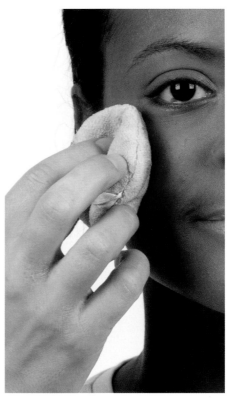

⊕ Normal or dry skin

For normal or dry skin, to set makeup lightly and control shine, dip your powder brush into loose powder, shake to remove excess product, and sweep over the T-zone first, then over the rest of the face from the forehead downward.

⊕ Oily skin

For oily skin or a longer-lasting finish, apply loose powder with a velour puff. To set the makeup and control shine, press the powder into the skin in a rolling motion, then do a second layer on the T-zone. The skin will not look too matte, as once the makeup settles, the natural oils in the skin will give it a dewy effect.

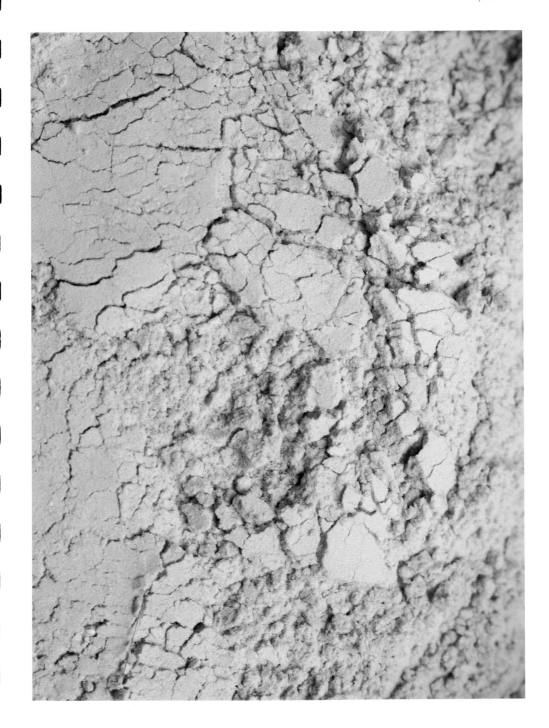

CONTOURING

With makeup, you can alter your face shape to give the illusion of a perfect, symmetrical face. Because an oval face shape is considered the ideal, you can use a combination of shading and highlighting on all other face shapes to make them appear more oval. You can also enhance or reduce the appearance of certain features. Shading and highlighting your features in this way is called contouring.

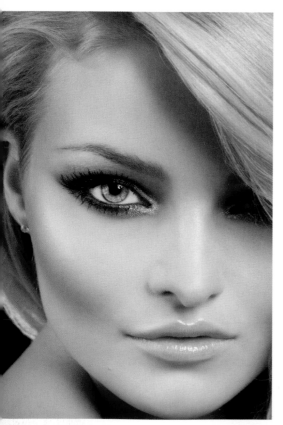

The easiest way to contour is to use matte powders, such as blush. You can also use foundation, which gives a very natural, subtle finish, or use cream blushes that have no shimmer in them. It is a difficult technique, which takes a lot of practice to do correctly.

Use contouring to play down your flaws:
Double chin Shade under the chin to minimize the appearance, using a shade two or three shades darker than your skin tone. Highlight on the tip of the chin and blend all edges well.
Wide or large nose For a wide nose, contour to minimize along both sides. If your nose is long, shade under the tip of the nose. If you dislike your nose it is a good idea to draw attention to another area of your face, such as the eyes or lips.
High or wide forehead For a high forehead, shade along the perimeter to visually reduce the height. If your forehead is wide and you would like to reduce its width, shade the temples.

To play up a feature such as cheekbones, use a paler shade of matte powder or foundation than your skin tone. To enhance cheekbones, apply along the top of the cheekbones. To make your eyes seem bigger, highlight under the brow bone.

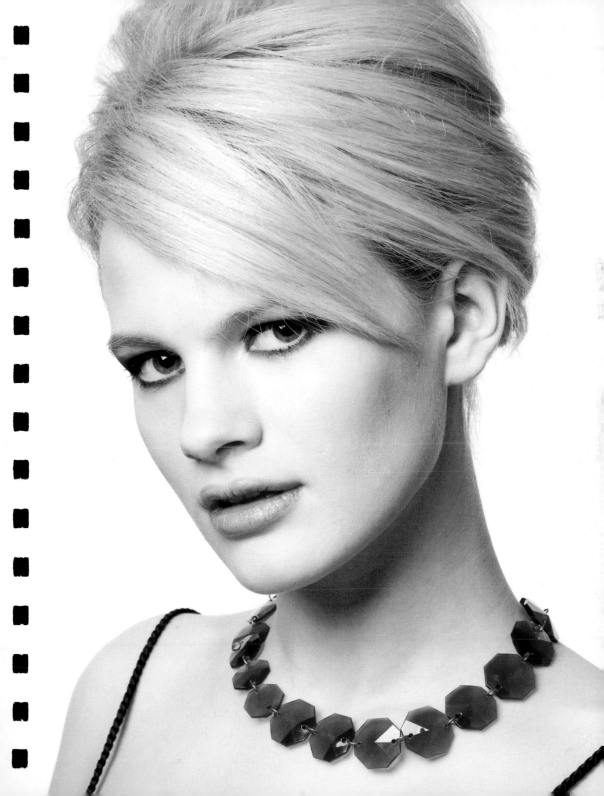

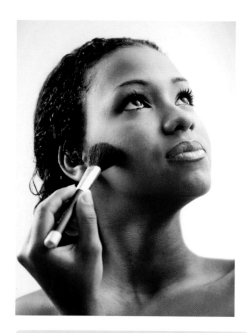

Shading and highlighting

Whether you choose to use powder or cream to enhance or play down your features and face shape, when you are contouring, the edges should be blended really well for a seamless, subtle effect.

Where to shade and highlight

1 Shading Shade under the cheekbone to add definition, create cheekbones where they are not visible, slim the face, and add depth.

2 Highlighting Highlight on top of the cheekbones to bring them forward. The highlight reflects light, making them appear higher and lifting the features.

3 Shading Shade the temples to soften a square face or make a wide forehead appear narrower.

4 Shading Contour the eye to add depth, shading along and slightly above the crease.

5 Highlighting and shading To alter the appearance of a wide nose, highlight the bridge vertically down the center, shade on either side of the nostrils, and add highlight on the cheeks directly next to the edge of the nostrils.

6 Highlighting To open, lift, or make eyes appear bigger, highlight on the brow bone under the arch of the eyebrow and on the inner corner of the eye.

7 Highlighting Highlight under the outer corner of the eye for instant lift and to waken tired eyes.

8 Shading To shorten a long nose, shade under the tip.

9 Highlighting To enhance the shape of the lips, highlight above the top lip along the bow and under the outer corners.

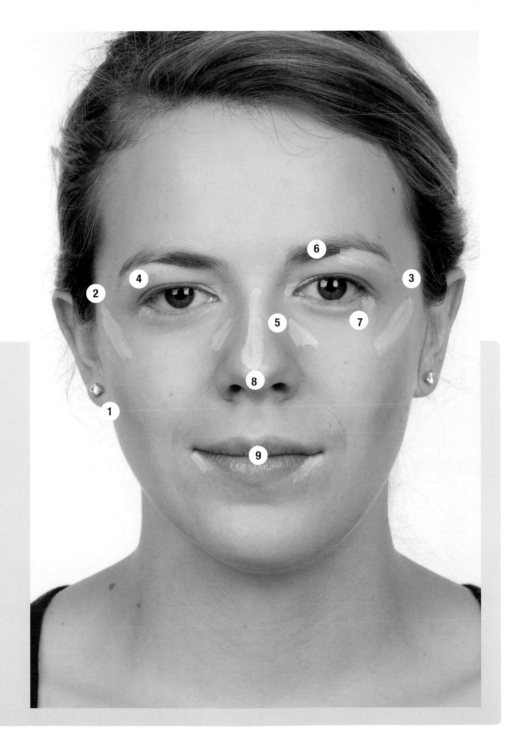

Basic contouring

All face shapes benefit from some basic contouring to enhance the features.

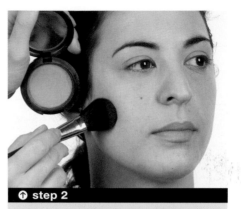

↑ step 2

Shade this area with a matte blush, first using a color one shade darker than the skin tone, then switching to one two shades darker than the skin tone if the effect is not visible enough. Blend the edges so they are invisible.

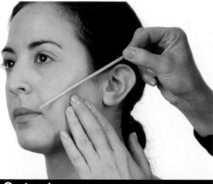

↑ step 1

To establish where to apply the shading, either use your fingers to feel the hollow of the cheek or, looking in a mirror, hold an orange stick, pen, or the handle of a makeup brush, against your face and line it up with the corner of your mouth and corner of the ear.

→ step 3

To narrow or give a more curved shape to the forehead, use shading. As a guide for where to apply the countour color on the temples, use the orange stick or another straight object. Make an imaginary line from the outer corner of the nose, through the outer corner of the eye, to the hairline. Shade above this line on the temple, making sure you blend the edges well.

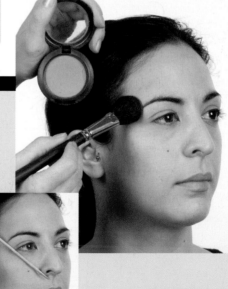

Contouring different face shapes

Round face

Contour a round face to make it seem more oval. Shade from the hollow of the cheek to the jawline along an imaginary line from the corner of the mouth to the top of the ear and the side of the forehead across the temple. A characteristic of a round face is plump cheeks, which hide the cheekbones, so use a darker shade of contour blush as it is harder to define this face shape.

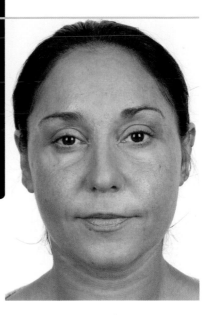

Square face

A square face has a solid jawline and unnoticeable cheekbones. To soften the jawline, contour under the cheekbone down to the jawline from the middle of the cheek back to the ear. Also contour the outer corners of the forehead above the temples, creating more of a rounded shape. To enhance cheekbones, highlight on top of them.

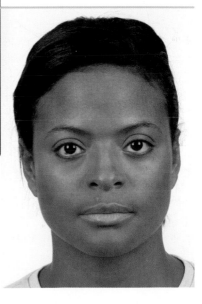

Long face

Apply contour powder or foundation two shades darker than the skin tone onto the forehead close to the hairline, under the cheekbones on the lower part of the cheeks, and across the bottom of the chin slightly above the jawline. Then apply blush directly on the cheekbones and highlight above the cheekbones and on the temples.

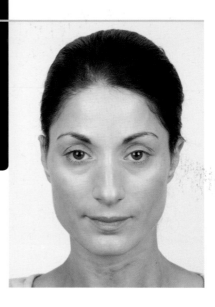

Heart-shaped face

Apply contour powder or foundation two shades darker than the skin tone to the temples and chin. Then apply highlighter to the lower cheeks on the jawline and blush directly on the cheekbones.

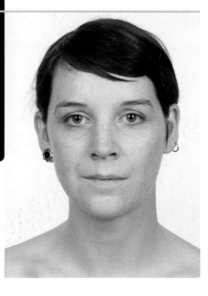

Pro Tip

Oval is considered to be the ideal face shape. To alter how your face appears, use a combination of contouring, highlighting, and clever blush placement.

- To contour, I would recommend using matte blush or foundation two shades darker than the skin tone.

- Highlighter can be either foundation that is two shades lighter than the skin tone; a matte powder, which could be a matte eyeshadow; or a cream highlighter.

- Always make sure that all the edges are blended well and there are no hard lines.

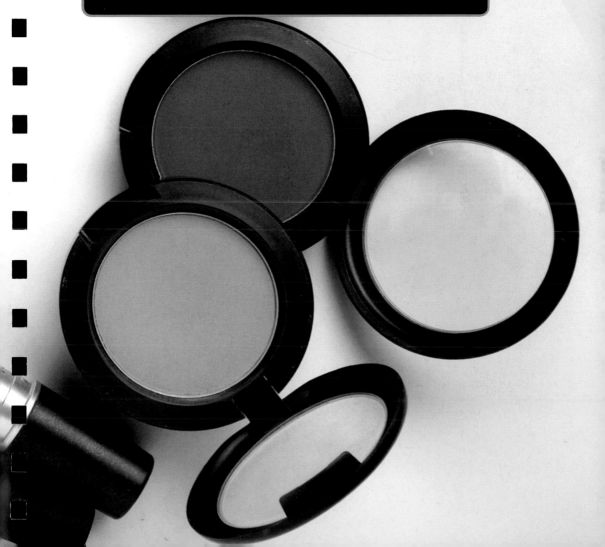

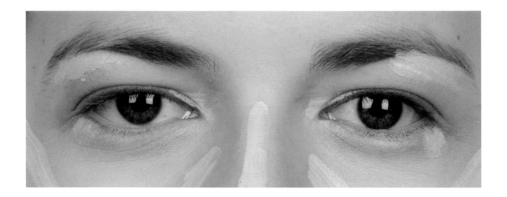

Contouring eyes

Contouring eyes is usually done with eyeshadow as part of an eye makeup routine. It can, however, be done with lighter and darker foundation or concealer. The picture above illustrates clearly where the darker and lighter colors should be used when making up eyes. Highlighter is applied under the arch of the eyebrow, on the inner corner of the eye, and under the outer corner. Shading is applied slightly above the socket line. All edges should be faded and blended into each other and the surrounding skin.

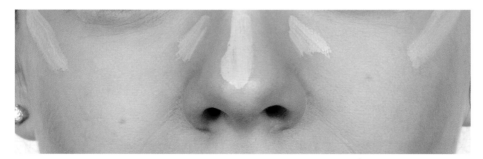

Contouring the nose

The most natural effect is achieved when you use cream products such as foundation or concealer, but it is possible to use matte powder blushes. Apply highlighter vertically on top of the bridge of the nose. Add a little bit of highlighter on either side of the nose, close to the nose. For a long nose or wide tip, you can shade under the end of the nose or on the nostrils.

Pro Tip

Make your eye makeup bold to draw attention away from a striking nose.

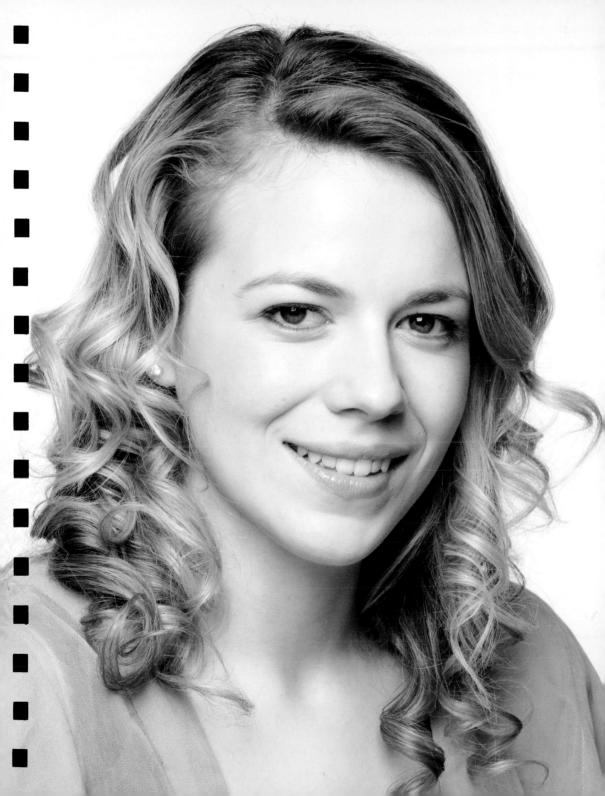

PRODUCTS FOR CHEEKS

Blush brightens your complexion and gives a healthy, youthful glow. It can be used to soften the shape of your face or to enhance features. There should be no hard edges to blush application; blending is key. The ideal blush should look like a natural flush of color.

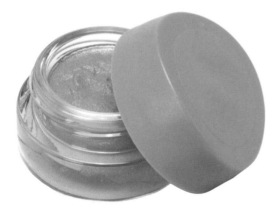

The density of blush products varies. It is better to have a highly pigmented product and apply it with a light touch than something wishy-washy that doesn't make an impact. Strong color blends in with natural skin tone.

Smiling at yourself in the mirror is quite useful to locate the apple of your cheeks, but don't smile when you actually apply blush as it can enhance fine lines and wrinkles. This is because smiling causes the skin to crease so there will be an uneven application of the blusher; when you stop smiling, the creases will still be visible.

If you have naturally red cheeks, don't dismiss blusher. Apply a tinted primer under your foundation and then assess how much of your redness shows through. You should be able to tone down the natural color and adjust with a blush to the shade you want.

FORMULATIONS

Blush comes in various formulations including cream, powder, or stain. There are various factors to consider when choosing which formula is best for you. You should take into account the texture of your skin and how you would like to apply the blush. The season may also be a factor; you may prefer a cream formula in the summer or after a vacation when you have a tan. A stain might be better when you are not using a foundation on vacation.

Powder

Works on most skin types and is easy to apply and blend. You need to have a powder brush to apply it and it should be used only on powdered skin. Even if your skin is just lightly dusted with translucent powder, it needs to have something on it, or blush won't blend, giving patchy results. Matte skin-toned powder blushes are used for contouring.

Stain

Good on younger, smooth skin; the finished look is sheer and long-lasting. Stains can be hard to blend and dry quickly, so you have to work fast. It can take some practice to get an even application. This formula works best with little or no foundation, so is especially suitable for the summer or when on vacation. Be careful; it will stain your fingers and clothes.

Cream

Is best suited to smooth skin and can be used on dry skin. Requires no tools or brushes to apply—it can be applied with fingers or a small fiber-optic brush. It goes on smoothly, and gives a dewy finish. It should be used only on unpowdered skin. It can take practice to get the blending right. It is hydrating, so it is suitable for dry or older skins and lasts longer than powder. Layering cream and then powder blush gives a long-lasting, strong effect.

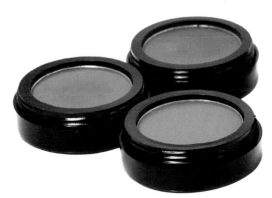

Gel

Gel blush is very sheer and adds a very natural glow to the skin. Gel blush is good for oily skin, as it is oil-free. Like a stain, gel blush is fast-drying, so it needs to be worked quickly. It can be used over foundation or on bare skin.

Bronzer

Used to imitate the glow you get from the sun. It should be applied on the high points of the face where the sun would naturally warm the color of the skin. It can be used to even out redness caused by rosacea. Bronzer is available in light, medium, or dark tones and can be gel, powder, or cream. Powder is easiest to use.

Shimmers

Shimmers are good for adding a light gleam to your face. They should be used sparingly and I would recommend them only at nighttime. You can apply shimmer on your cheekbones, forehead, and in the bow of your upper lip.

Selection

Although most skin tones can wear most colors, knowing what suits you, using the right product, and applying it correctly, will give you the most flattering look and make you more confident to experiment.

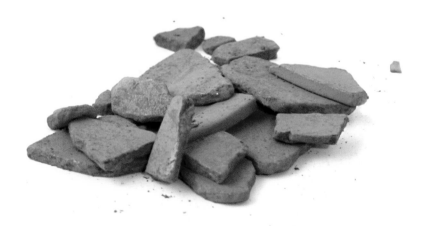

20s

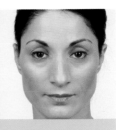

Do

- Go for a dewy look; let your natural youthful radiance show.
- Choose fresh pinks.
- Try gels and stains as these work best over little foundation and this is an age when you are not likely to need much.
- Try blush with a bit of shimmer to give the skin a sheen.
- Use dual-purpose products such as creamy blush that doubles as a lip product.

Don't

- Use a stain if your skin is not smooth; it will highlight bumps.
- Wear too much blusher.
- Apply highlighter if you have bumpy skin or acne.

30s

Do

- To keep a youthful glow, use highlighter on the bridge of your nose, cheekbones, and forehead.
- For a natural flush, use a pink cream blush on the apples of your cheeks. For radiance use a soft, slightly shimmery bronzer.
- Try layering cream and powder blush for a look that lasts all day.
- Play up your smooth skin; hopefully acne is behind you.

Don't

- Go for colors with a purple/blue undertone as they will be aging.
- Forget to blend the edges of blush well; stripes are not a good look.

40s

Do

- Use blush to give your face a fresher, brighter look.
- Try cream blusher.
- Have a blush shade for summer and one for winter.
- Use matte bronzer for warmth.
- Cover any redness with foundation and apply subtle blush on top.
- Remember bronzer can tone down redness.

Don't

- Use the same shade of blush you used in your 20s.
- Be afraid to try new products and formulas.
- Overdo the highlighter; it will accentuate fine lines.

50s

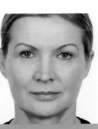

Do

- Use an illuminating primer.
- Use a bronzer for a healthy, sun-kissed look.
- Look objectively at your skin tone and adjust blush color to suit.
- Try cream blush.
- Invest in good-quality blush products; the intensity of pigment will give a better finish.

Don't

- Overcompensate for a paler, gray-tinged complexion by applying too much blush.
- Apply blush in one direction, whether it is cream or powder; blend it in small circles.
- Contour too heavily.
- Apply highlighter; use an illuminating primer for sheen.

Blush application

Blush is used for a variety of effects including narrowing a wide face, and sharpening, defining, lifting, and softening features. The ways in which blush is used in each of these situations varies slightly.

Softening features

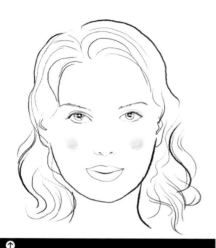

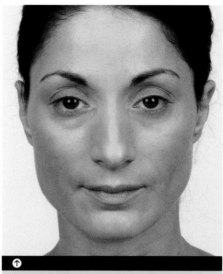

⬆
Placing blush on the apples of the cheeks softens an angular face and will accentuate freshness.

⬆
To locate the apples of your cheeks, smile. Place a finger on the highest point and when you stop smiling, check this hasn't dropped too far toward your mouth. If it does drop considerably, place the blush above this point. If your finger remains high, place blush in this place. Circle your finger or brush outward as you apply the blush, lifting and blending up along the cheekbone, blending the edges of the blush well.

Lifting features

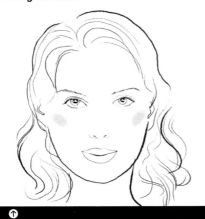

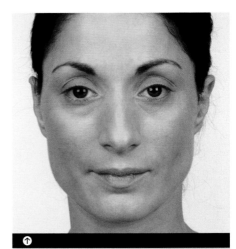

⬆ To accentuate good cheekbones, to give the impression of having them, or to give the face a lift, apply blush high on the cheekbones near the eyes.

⬆ Use your fingers to locate the top of your cheekbone. Apply blush along the top of the cheekbone from the middle of the cheek upward. To blend, make small circles along the cheekbone, circling upward and outward as you blend toward the eye.

Sharpening features

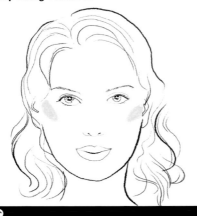

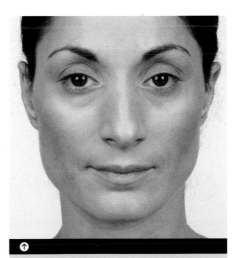

⬆ For a sophisticated appearance, especially on a round face to make it more angular. Apply just on the underside of the cheekbone, not too low down.

⬆ Use your fingers to locate your cheekbone and feel for the underside. Be careful not to go too low. The line of unblended blush will slant from the ear toward the corner of the mouth. Smudge the line and blend the edges well.

Narrowing features

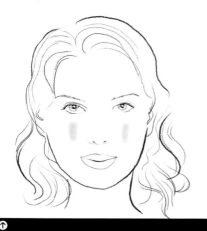

⬆

Placing blush in a vertical line on either side of the nose will slim a wide face.

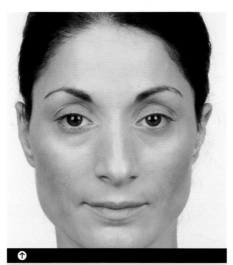

⬆

Smile to locate the center of the apples of the cheeks. Leave your finger where it is and stop smiling. Your finger will move toward your nose. This will tell you how far from your nose to apply the blush. Apply blush along this line from the bottom of the cheekbone to just past the end of the nose. Smudge the blush and blend the edges.

Pro Tip

To take the attention away from a wide nose, place blush wide on your face, farther away from your nose. To reduce the length of a long face, place blush horizontally from the center of the apples of the cheeks toward the ears, and blend.

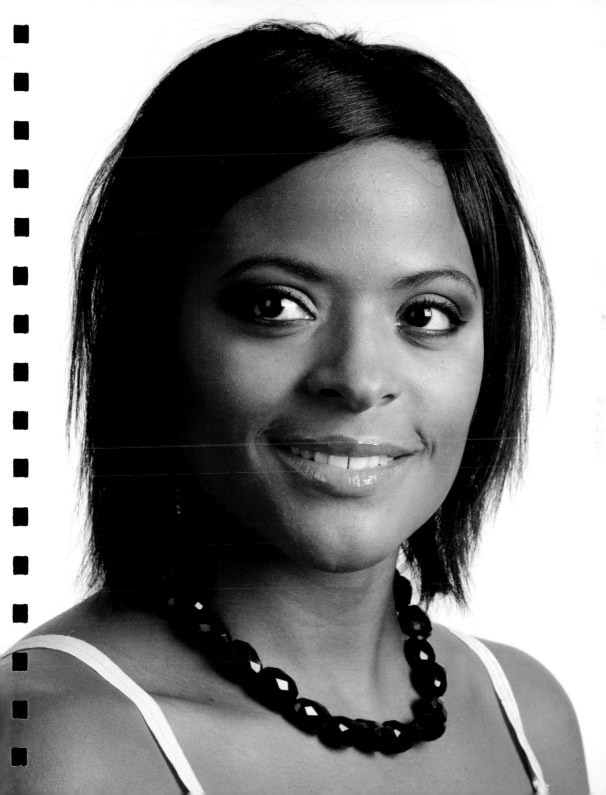

LIPS

Most women know how to apply lipstick. It is the most straightforward of all makeup to use and can be applied in seconds. Lips are central to the overall look of the face. The choice of lip color should balance and be in harmony with all the other makeup; you can create a makeup look based around your choice of lip color, but it should always be the last thing applied.

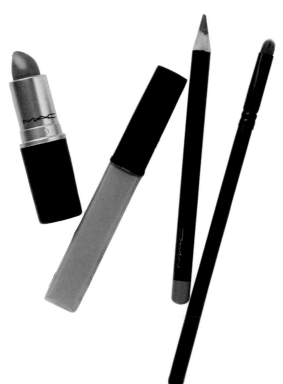

I believe that with the huge range of shades available in beauty salons and drugstores, there is something in each color group to suit everyone. Test a range of tones to establish whether you suit cool or warm undertones and go for shades with this undertone. If you are testing lip colors and can't try them on your lips, test them on your fingertip, as fingertips have more red in them and therefore are closer to your lip color than the back of your hand. Darker colors can make small lips look smaller; equally light colors, especially glossy ones, make lips appear fuller.

It is important to look after your lips. Lips that are soft and well cared for will look better with lip products on them. Lips do not have sebaceous glands to produce natural oil, so they can easily become dry and cracked. Exfoliate and moisturize with lip balm regularly, just as you would the rest of your face.

Besides a huge choice of colors, there are also a bewildering number of textures and formulas on the market, as cosmetic companies come out with new ones each year.

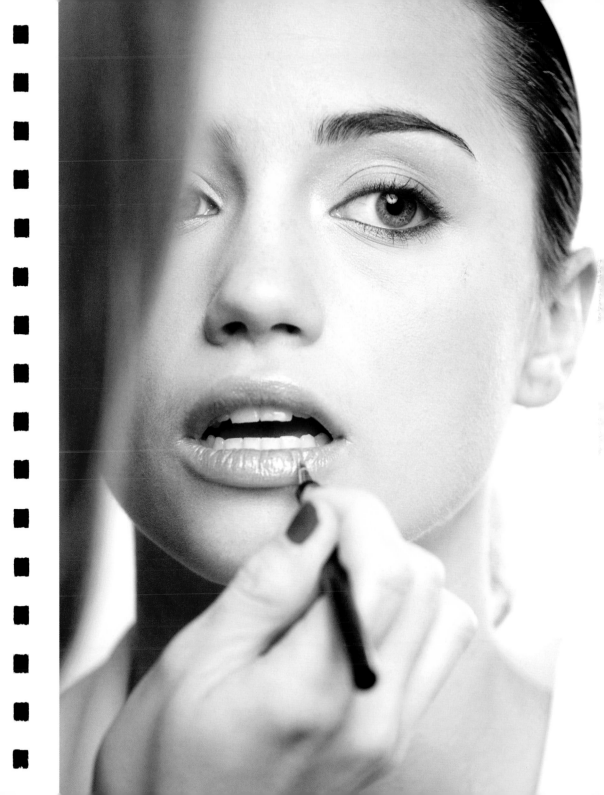

Formulations

Lipliner

Defines the lips, and increases the longevity of the lipstick. New formulas are creamier, making them easier to use than traditional drier ones.

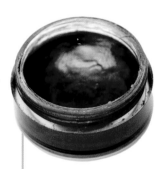

Stain

Long-lasting and highly pigmented. Usually comes with its own brush for application. Can last for up to six hours but dries quickly and can be hard to wipe off if you make a mistake.

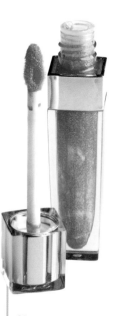

Gloss

Comes with its own applicator so is very portable. Can be clear, tinted, or colored. Some glosses are specifically formulated to be plumping. Gives lips shine and makes them look fuller.

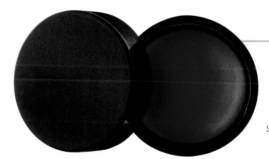

Tinted balm

Good if you don't like lipstick or glosses. Helps to soften and moisturize the lips and gives a sheer wash of color.

Selection

When you are wearing no makeup, choose a nude lipstick shade that will match the natural color of your lips. Do not go for a nude color that is paler than your natural lips; it will make you look pasty and unwell.

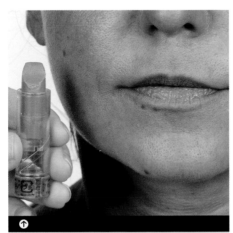

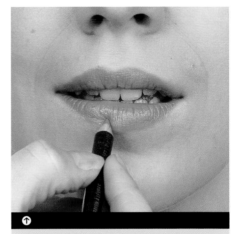

Hold the lipstick up to your face in good light, when you are wearing minimal makeup, and your hair is pulled off your face. Apply the lipstick with a brush, to work it into the lips, and blot firmly over the lipstick with your finger.

Pink can be flattering on anyone; you just need to find the right shade of pink to suit you. Apply lipstick in a soft pink. Then to define the lips and to prevent the lipstick sliding off, lightly apply lip pencil on top of the lipstick. Apply clear gloss on top for a fresh natural look or use a tinted gloss for more intensity.

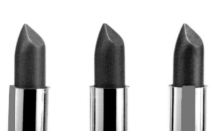

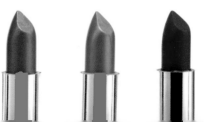

Applying lip color

For a long-lasting, defined look, use lipliner, lipstick, and then a touch of gloss. Filling the whole lip with the pencil will ensure an even application of color and increase the longevity of the color without the dry look of a matte lipstick.

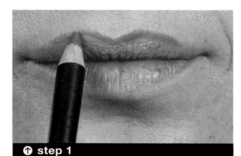

⬆ step 1

Line the lips with a pencil that matches the natural color of the lips; start with the top lip, drawing toward the center, keeping the line on the natural line of the lip.

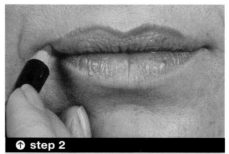

⬆ step 2

Keep working toward the center, working the pencil from farther out toward the center of the lips.

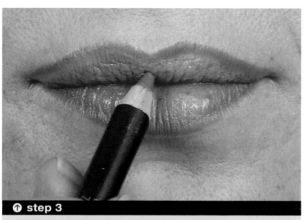

⬆ step 3

Apply the lipliner along the bottom lip, first drawing the line on the middle of the lip and then from the corners toward the middle. Fill in the whole lip area with the pencil.

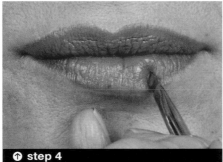

↑ step 4

Work matching lipstick into the lips with a lip brush, pressing the lipstick into the lips.

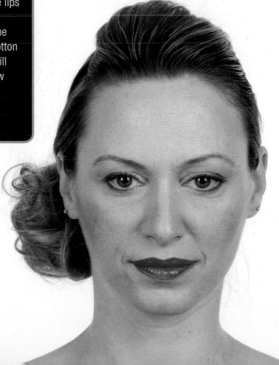

↑ step 5

Blot, then apply clear gloss with a lip brush in the center of the lips.

Pro Tip

To enhance the strength of the lip line and stop lipstick from bleeding, apply concealer around the outside of the lips up to the lip line.

If you smudge your lipstick or the line goes wrong, clean up with a cotton swab dipped in cleanser and then fill the hole with concealer and re-draw the line.

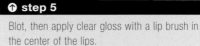
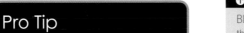

Exaggerating lip shapes

The natural lip shape can be altered or exaggerated by applying lipliner and lipstick in different ways to enhance and disguise.

Cupid's bow

Start at the top and draw half a circle one side at a time inside the natural lip line from the outside edge toward the middle. Stand back as you work to check that the sides are equal. These lips are smaller than your normal lips so you will need to decide on the point where they will finish. Mark this with a dot on both sides before lining the bottom lip, starting in the middle and drawing outward a bit at a time.

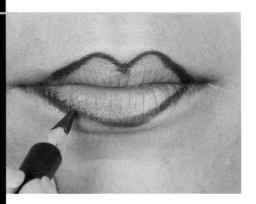

Full

Outline a cupid's bow (see above), just outside the natural lip line. Working from the outside in, join the edges of the top lip up to the cupid's bow. Draw in the middle of the bottom lip just outside the natural lip line. Draw from the outside edges to join in the middle.

Pro Tip

Rest your hand on a velour puff to steady it when applying lipliner. Fill in with a pencil to create a long-lasting base before applying lipstick on top.

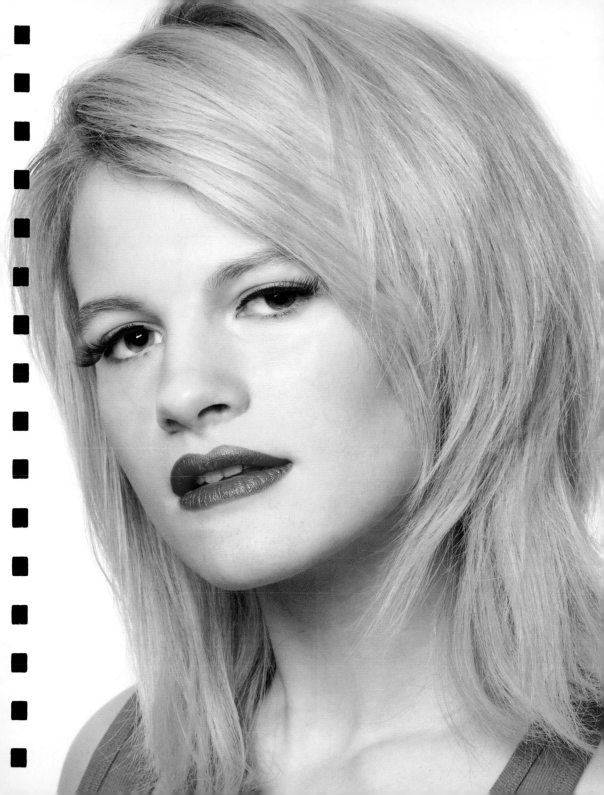

EYES

Your eyes are just one component of the makeup you apply on a daily basis, but it is the key component, and the one on which you will probably spend most time. It pays to take your time in getting to know the basics—you will use these techniques again and again and they will become second nature. Being able to do a basic eye makeup well will give you the confidence to do any eye makeup look you desire.

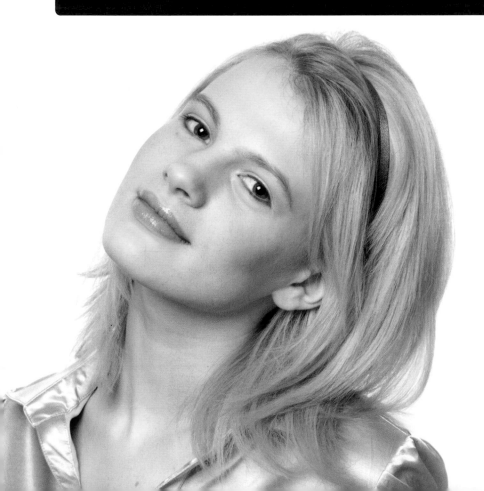

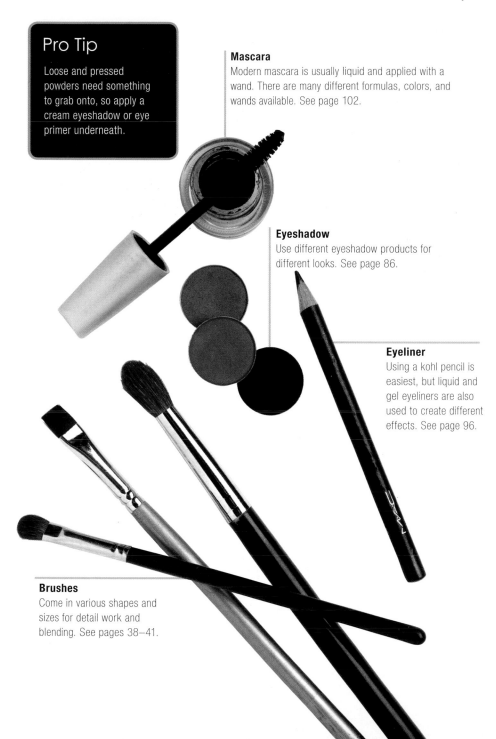

Pro Tip

Loose and pressed powders need something to grab onto, so apply a cream eyeshadow or eye primer underneath.

Mascara

Modern mascara is usually liquid and applied with a wand. There are many different formulas, colors, and wands available. See page 102.

Eyeshadow

Use different eyeshadow products for different looks. See page 86.

Eyeliner

Using a kohl pencil is easiest, but liquid and gel eyeliners are also used to create different effects. See page 96.

Brushes

Come in various shapes and sizes for detail work and blending. See pages 38–41.

EYESHADOW

Just like lipstick and blusher, there are many different types of eyeshadow products available.

1 Pressed powder

The most common type of eyeshadow and easiest to use. Pressed eyeshadow comes in every color imaginable and with a variety of finishes from matte to glittery. Powder is long-wearing and colors blend well together.

2 Loose shimmer balls

These have stronger color pigments or shimmer than pressed powder for a more intense look. Some brands have pure pigment powders, which give a really strong result and can be used anywhere on the face. Loose balls and powders can be messy to use, so always do the eyes first and give yourself plenty of time.

3 Cream eyeshadow

Comes in various packaging including compact and tube, and is very easy to spread over the eyelid with a fingertip for an instant wash of color. Cream eyeshadows can crease easily, so the eyelid should be prepped with a thin layer of foundation and the eyeshadow should be set by pressing powder on top. Cream to powder eyeshadows go on creamy but dry to a powder finish. They are very long-wearing and make an excellent eye base.

4 Creamy powder

This product is easy to apply and comes in a range of textures. It is long-wearing and makes an excellent eye base.

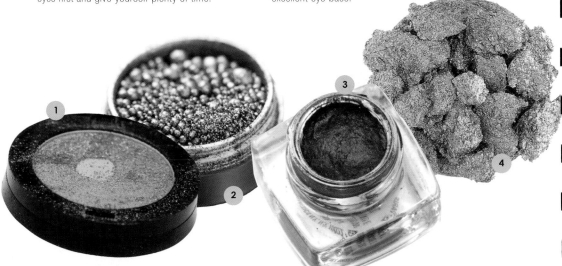

Pro Tip

It is a good idea to accumulate a set of eyeshadow brushes so you can keep different brushes to use with neutral, medium, and dark eyeshadows.

Eyeshadow application

Learn the steps for basic eye makeup application and everything else will follow. You can adapt these steps for any color, enhance them for a more smoky look, or use lighter colors for a more natural look—the principles remain the same.

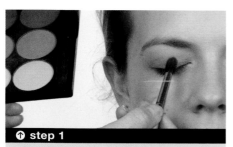

↑ step 1

First apply foundation lightly over the whole eyelid area to act as a base, even out skin tone, and cover any discoloration. The skin over the eyelid is very thin so veins and discoloration can show through. Apply nude/beige matte eyeshadow over the whole lid area to set foundation and form a barrier against natural oils that can cause eyeshadow to crease. It also acts as a blending base for other colors applied on top. Use a clean dome-shaped eyeshadow blending brush.

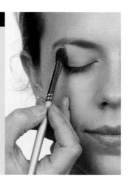

➜ step 2

Apply a lighter eyeshadow, blending well under the arch of the eyebrow and on the inner corner of the eye.

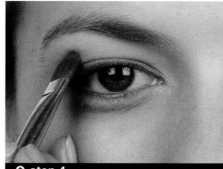

➜ step 3

With a smaller eyeshadow brush, apply matte taupe eyeshadow on the outer third of the eyelid from the lash line, blending inward and upward into the crease of the eyelid.

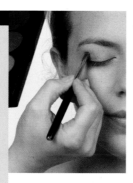

↑ step 4

With the eye open, take the taupe eyeshadow slightly above the crease and blend the edges well, making a circular motion with your wrist. For a natural look you could stop here, finishing the look with mascara.

Pro Tip

Cream eyeshadows make a good base for loose pigments or glitter.

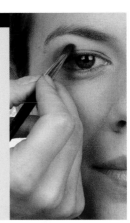

→ step 6

With your eye open as before, blend the darker color slightly above the crease, smudging the edges with circular movements of the wrist so that they fade seamlessly.

↑ step 5

To build on this and make the eye smokier, brush the taupe eyeshadow inward so it covers two-thirds of the eyelid. Blend a dark matte brown over the outer third of the eyelid from the lashes into the crease.

→ step 7

With a fine detail eyeshadow brush, apply matte black eyeshadow along the top and bottom lash lines close to the root of the lashes. To finish, curl the lashes and apply mascara.

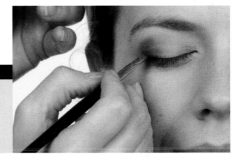

Pro Tip

If you are getting married and want your eye makeup to last all day, apply a nude cream to powder as an eye base and then build up the eye look with powder eyeshadows.

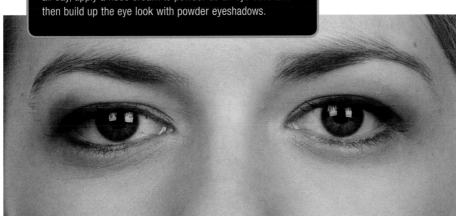

EYELASHES

Your eyelashes open, accentuate, and frame the eye. Long eyelashes are considered a sign of femininity in many cultures.

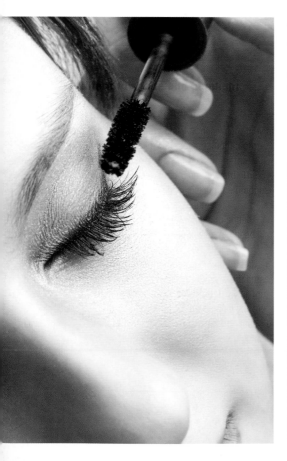

You can work with your own lashes, curling and coating them with mascara, or you can boost your natural lashes with false ones. If your lashes are sparse and you don't want to use false lashes, smudging liner or eyeshadow into the root of the lashes will give the illusion of a thicker lash line.

Eyelash facts

- We have eyelashes to protect our eyes from debris. They are the body's warning system if an alien object is approaching the eye.
- If your eyelashes are pulled out, they will take approximately seven to eight weeks to grow back.
- The lifespan of an eyelash is approximately 150–200 days.
- The average number of eyelashes is 150–200 on the top eyelid and 75–100 on the bottom.

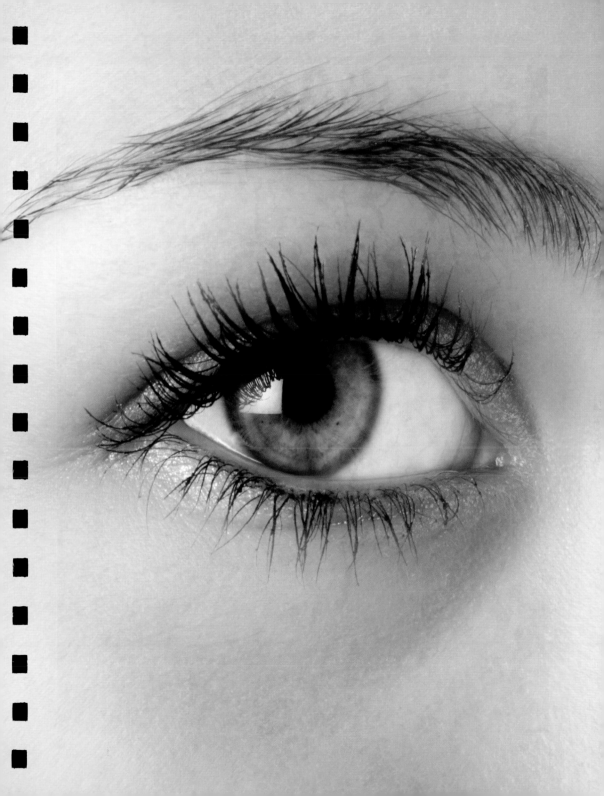

False eyelashes

Eyelashes fall into three categories: individual, half set, and full set. There are many variations on the following:

Full set, full impact These lashes are suitable for large or Asian eyes. Avoid if your eyes are small or your natural lashes are sparse. They come in half or full set. Half lashes are glued to the outer half of the eyelid and are easier to apply than a full set, but sometimes the effect can be unbalancing if it isn't continued all the way along the lash line.

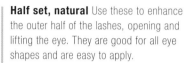

Half set, natural Use these to enhance the outer half of the lashes, opening and lifting the eye. They are good for all eye shapes and are easy to apply.

Full set, natural A step up from the half set, they are suitable for any eye shape. Harder to apply than a half set. They need to be measured against the width of your lash line and trimmed if too long.

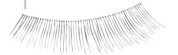

Full set, medium impact These lashes are good for a full-impact effect on sparse lashes. The lashes crisscross to give maximum density without being too heavy. They will need to be measured and trimmed if too long.

Individual, bunches Suit all eye shapes and look very natural, but can be tricky to glue to sparse natural lashes. They come in short, medium, and long so you can tailor the effect to suit the length of your lashes and the impact you want them to make.

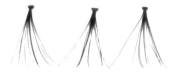

Individual, singles These give a natural effect, enhancing your own eyelash hairs, but they are hard to use. It is tricky to get them to sit in the right direction; if your natural lashes are sparse, there is not much to glue them to. They do not enhance lash density.

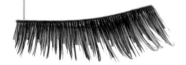

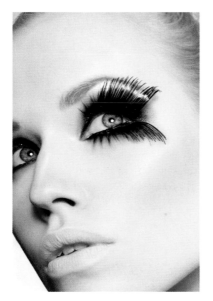

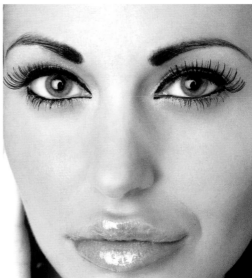

Pro Tip

Eyelashes are attached to the eyes with glue. If you are a false eyelash addict, it is worth investing in some surgical adhesive from a professional makeup supplier. This glue is more elastic than the glue that comes with the lashes, it lasts longer, and the lashes come away with less pulling.

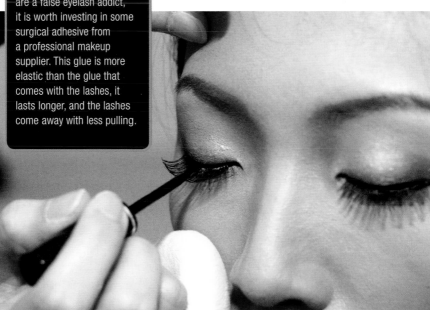

False eyelash application

Eyelashes are the final element of your eye makeup. To make it easier to blend the lash band of a full or half set, apply eyeliner along your top lash line before and, if necessary, again once you have applied the eyelashes.

Individual

◯ step 1

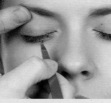

Put a dollop of glue on the back of your hand or on a palette. Once it has become tacky, pick up the lash with tweezers and dip the end of the lash into the glue. Apply the lash as close to the root of your natural lashes as possible, dropping it into place and then pushing into the root and holding for a few seconds.

◯ step 2

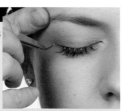

With individual lashes you can use the different lengths to thicken your own lashes or to add natural-looking additional length and thickness all the way along. Here I have applied shorter lashes on the inside, medium-length ones in the middle, and the longest ones on the outer corner.

Half set

◯ step 1

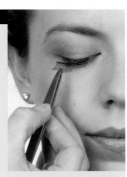

Pick the lash up with tweezers and apply glue all the way along the lash band. I find it easier and less messy to apply the glue directly onto the lashes, rather than pulling lashes through glue placed on a palette or the back of your hand. Wait for the glue to become tacky and then drop on top of the natural lashes as close to the root as possible.

◯ step 2

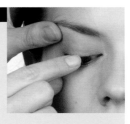

With your finger, move the lashes into place and push down into the root. Hold for a few seconds. Once the glue has dried, lightly apply a thin coat of mascara to blend them with your natural lashes.

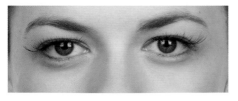

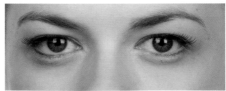

Full set

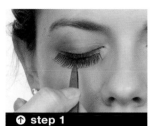

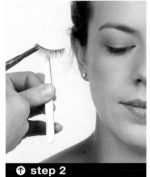

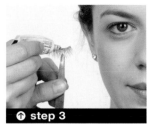

↑ step 1

Pick the lashes up with tweezers and measure the length against the eyelid.

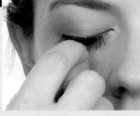

↑ step 2

Trim the outer ends of the lashes to fit the width of the eyelid.

↑ step 3

Apply glue all the way along the lash band. It is easier and less messy to apply the glue directly onto the lashes.

→ step 4

I find it easiest to hold the full lashes between my thumb and forefinger to put the lash band in place on the natural lashes. The lash band should sit against the root of the natural lashes.

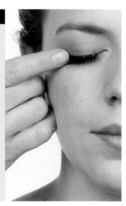

→ step 5

Push the lashes into place, tapping all along the lash band. Open your eye and look in the mirror, and make sure there isn't a gap between the natural lashes and false lashes.

→ step 6

Once the glue has dried, apply a thin coat of mascara to blend your natural lashes and the false lashes together (see page 102).

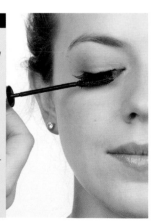

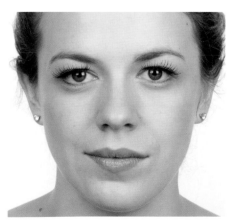

EYELINER

Different types of eyeliner are widely available, from your local drugstore to beauty supply stores. How each kind is applied varies according to the type of product and the effect you are trying to achieve.

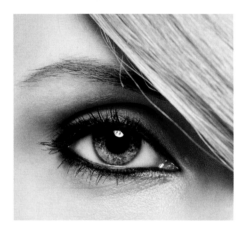

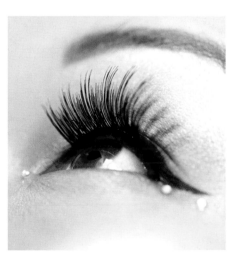

Pro Tips

- To wing eyeliner from the outer corner, first line along lashes and then flick wrist up and away from the outer corner, making short strokes and lengthening the line a little bit at a time.
- If you use kohl pencil eyeliner on the inside of the lower eyelid but find it runs downward, brush a dark matte powder eyeshadow under the bottom lashes to act as a barrier and help keep eyeliner in place.
- Don't line all the way around the eye if you have small eyes; it will make them look even smaller.
- Colored liquid eyeliners can be smudged over the eyelid and used as an eye base. They will make bright-colored eyeshadow even more vibrant.
- If you draw a strong liquid line along the top lashes, either leave the underneath bare or softly define; anything too harsh will draw the eyes down.
- Liquid eyeliner is effective when re-creating a period look.

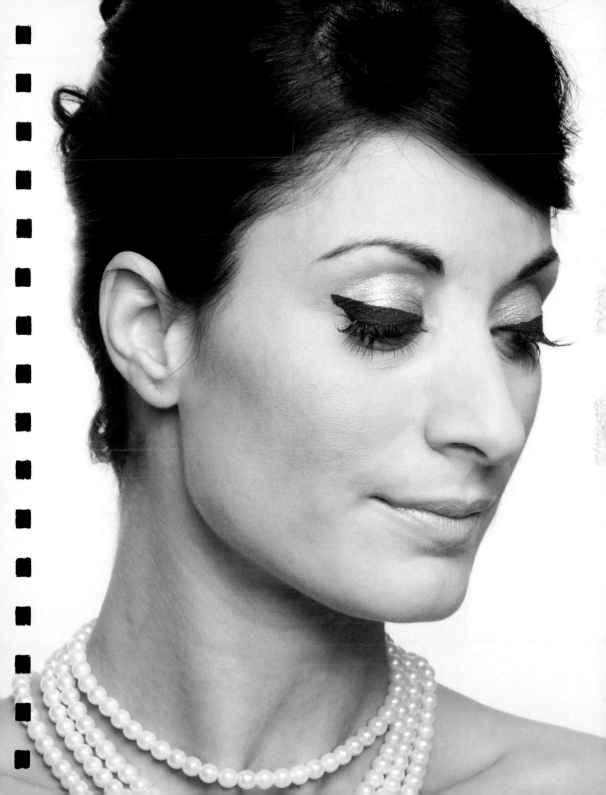

Eyeliner application

Eyeliner adds definition and impact to the lash line. It can be used to complement an eye look or as an eye look in itself.

Applying eyeliner requires a steady hand. If it goes wrong, you can use a cotton swab to smudge the line into your eyeshadow and try again, or alter your eye look slightly to suit the smudged line! If you aren't confident, use powder eyeshadow to start off with. Liquid liner is the hardest to apply and is only for the seasoned pro!

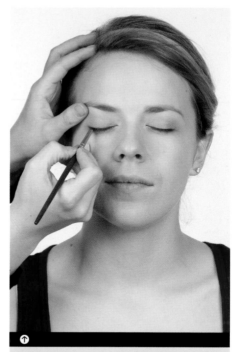

When applying eyeliner, it helps to pull your eyelid taught so the skin doesn't ruffle, creating a broken line. Draw the line in one direction; once it is all the way across the lid, go over it in the other direction. Eyeliner is usually applied after eyeshadow and before mascara.

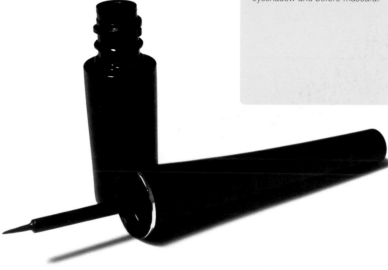

Applying powder eyeshadow

For softly defined eyes, line along the top and bottom lashes with eyeshadow. To give impact, use dark browns, blacks, and dark gray. The eyeshadow should be applied with a detail eye brush close to the roots of the upper and lower lashes.

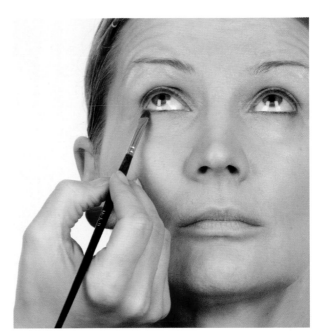

Applying pencil eyeliner

The texture of your eyeliner pencil should be soft and creamy; if it is too hard and dry, it will be very difficult to apply. To draw an eyeline with a pencil, first make sure it is freshly sharpened and then make short strokes in a line from the outside corner inward. Each small stroke should slightly overlap the end of the previous stroke. If your eyelids are loose and crepey, go over the line in the other direction to ensure it is unbroken. To apply kohl inside the lower eyelid, pull the lower lid down and draw from the outer corner inward.

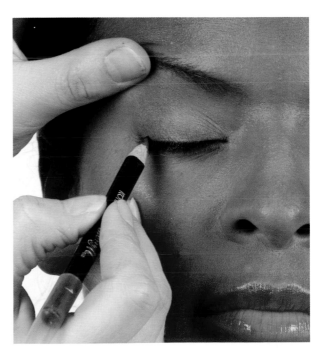

Applying cream or gel eyeliner

This liner comes in a pot and is applied with a brush. I prefer to use a flat liner brush but you could also use a fine tip angled liner brush. Using a flat liner brush means you don't have to drag the brush across the lid. Dip the brush in the product and then, starting at the outer corner, press the brush onto the lid and wiggle it slightly, then pull the brush away and move inward so you are slightly overlapping, and repeat. Using a fine detail brush, make small strokes as you would with a pencil, working from the outer corner inward.

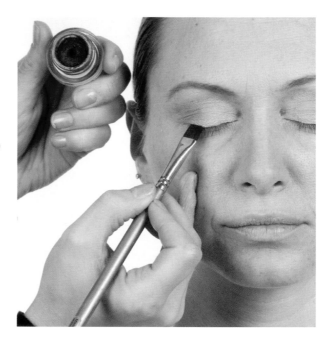

Applying liquid eyeliner

Liquid liner is good for re-creating period looks, or for when you want a visible solid line. It dries quickly, which makes it harder to use. The liner comes with its own applicator, which has a firm tip. Wipe the applicator after you have removed it from the liquid to remove clumps and then line the eyes from the outer corner inward. For a period look, build up the width of the line toward the outer corner and extend the line beyond the corner of the eye, flicking it upward.

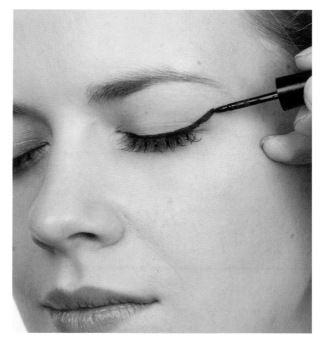

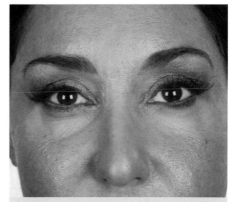

Eyeliner adds definition to the eyes and a professional finish to a day or bridal look.

Eyeliner is used to blend the lash band of false eyelashes into the natural lash line and eyeshadow.

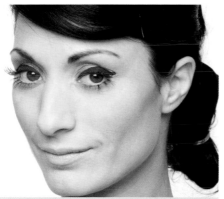

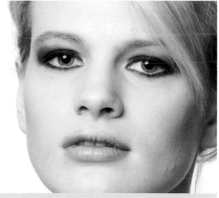

Eyeliner was popular in the 1950s and 1960s and can be used to give a retro feel to a makeup look.

Eyeliner is an essential component to a smoky eye look. It is used to blend the eyeshadow seamlessly into the root of the eyelashes, as well as to add intensity to a look.

MASCARA

Mascara was invented in the nineteenth century by Eugene Rimmel. Modern mascara was invented by a pharmacist in 1913 for his sister who was called Mabel and who later went on to form Maybelline. Waterproof mascara and the tube and wand applicator that are now so popular were both invented by Helena Rubenstein in the 1950s. Most women wear mascara every day—it is used to enhance lashes and draw attention to them. For women with fair lashes or pale coloring, mascara is essential.

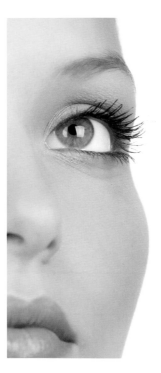

The majority of modern mascara is liquid and applied with a wand. In the past, cake mascara was popular, and it was applied with a comb. There are many different formulas, colors, and wands available. Wands can be straight, curved, or cone-shaped amongst others, and formulas can be thickening and defining. See page 104 for different types of mascara wand and their effects.

The way in which you apply mascara makes a huge difference; It should be applied right from the root to the tip in one or two coats.

Pro Tip

Apply a second coat of mascara when the first coat is almost but not completely dry. Adding another coat on top of totally dry mascara can make the first coat crumble.

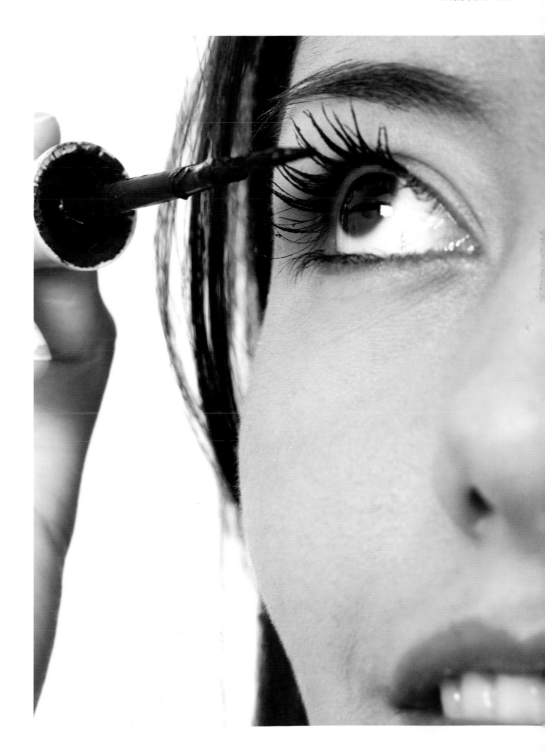

Mascara wand types and effects

Thickening

- Good for fine lashes, adds fibers, and makes lashes denser.
- Not as good for a daytime look as it can be clumpy.
- If used on both top and bottom lashes on small eyes, it can make them appear even smaller.

Comb

- Separates lashes for a more natural day look.
- Good for fair or thin lashes as you can easily get right to the roots.
- Not suitable for thickening.

Fine detail

- Great for bottom lashes.
- Good for thin lashes and the finer hairs found toward the inner corner of the eye.
- Can add definition to the eyes.

Cone-shaped

- Most common type of brush.
- Great for any lash and makeup look.
- Can shape and define the eyes.
- Suitable for top and bottom lashes.
- The cone shape enables you to get a natural look, reaching the finer lashes toward the inner corner of the eye.

Full cone-shaped

- Good for widening eyes.
- Gives thick application of mascara and therefore thickens lashes.
- Suitable for evening/smoky eyes.
- Not suitable for bottom lashes.

Pro tips

- Replace your mascara often. It can be a breeding ground for bacteria and cause infection.
- Don't pump the brush in and out of the tube, the trapped air will dry the mascara out.
- Before your mascara is completely dry, comb the lashes through with a clean wand after you have applied the mascara to remove clumps.
- If your mascara smudges onto your eyelid or cheek, remove it with a cotton swab to disturb as little of your makeup as possible.

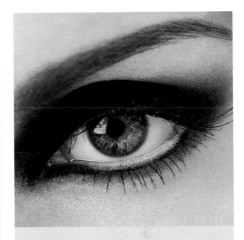

Turn the wand vertically to apply mascara to the bottom lashes. This will mean they won't clump together. Mascara on the bottom lashes should be applied in one coat only.

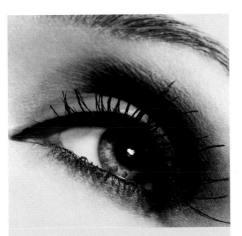

Even if you have long lashes, curl them to open up the eye. Apply one coat of mascara only, as two will make them too heavy. Apply right from the root, moving the wand from side to side as you move toward the tips.

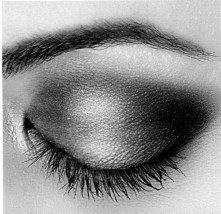

If you have short lashes and want to lengthen and thicken them, apply a coat of mascara on the top of the lashes first and then apply a coat on the underside.

Applying mascara

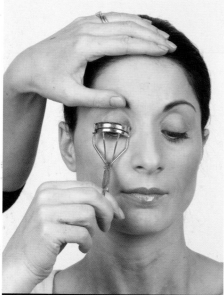

⬆ step 1

Apply mascara after you have completed your eye makeup. First curl your eyelashes, making sure the curler is as close to the root of the lash as possible; but before you squeeze the curler, ensure you only have hairs and no skin! I recommend curling the lashes on each eye twice.

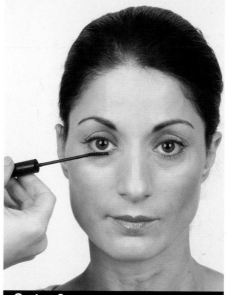

⬆ step 2

Place the mascara wand horizontally close to the root of the lash and massage it against the roots. Then wiggle it from side to side as you draw it toward the tips. Turn the wand vertically and separate the lashes all the way along the lid. Once the mascara on the top lashes has almost dried you can apply mascara on the bottom lashes. Apply mascara on the bottom lightly to avoid clumps and smudging the skin underneath.

Pro Tip

For a curled effect, first squeeze the lashes at the root with the eyelash curler, then release and squeeze two or three times more along the length of the lashes, working toward the tips. As you move away from the root, gradually turn your wrist so the curler is rotating away from the face.

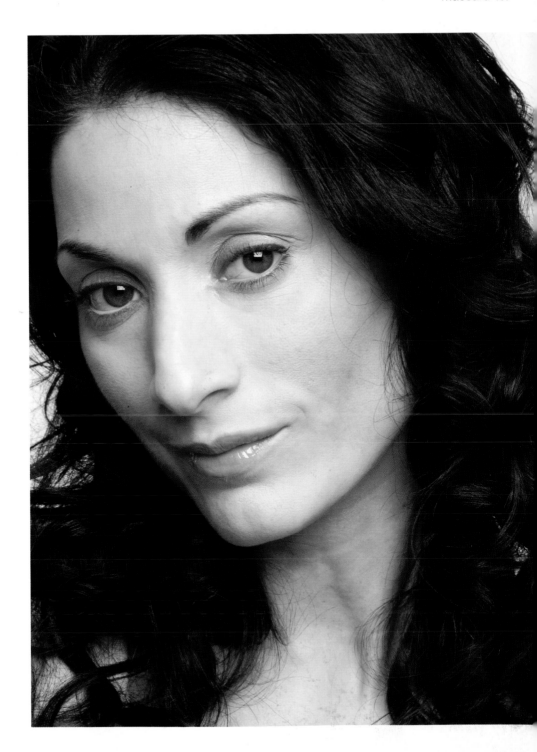

EYEBROWS

Your eyebrows add strength and definition to your face and frame your eyes, so they should be beautifully groomed. Reshaping your brows will transform your face. This can be done with tweezers, waxing, or threading or simply with brow powder, pencil, mascara, or gel. Eyebrows can also be darkened or lightened with dye.

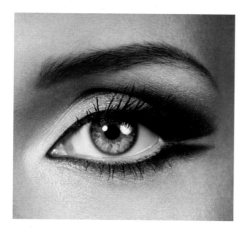

Scars and gaps in your eyebrows can be covered or filled. If you have nonexistent brows, don't panic. You can achieve natural results with pencil and powder. It is even possible to get an eyebrow wig where real hair is woven onto lace. I would never advise eyebrow tattooing—the effect is very unnatural and irreversible.

You can fill and reshape your brows with powder or an eyebrow pencil. Pencil is applied directly—make sure it has a good point and draw short feathery strokes, starting at the inner edge. Powder is applied with a slanted eyebrow brush, again with short feathery strokes, working from the inner corner outward.

Pro Tip

If your brows are really thin, you can fill them to look slightly thicker, but don't go overboard as the results will look unnatural.

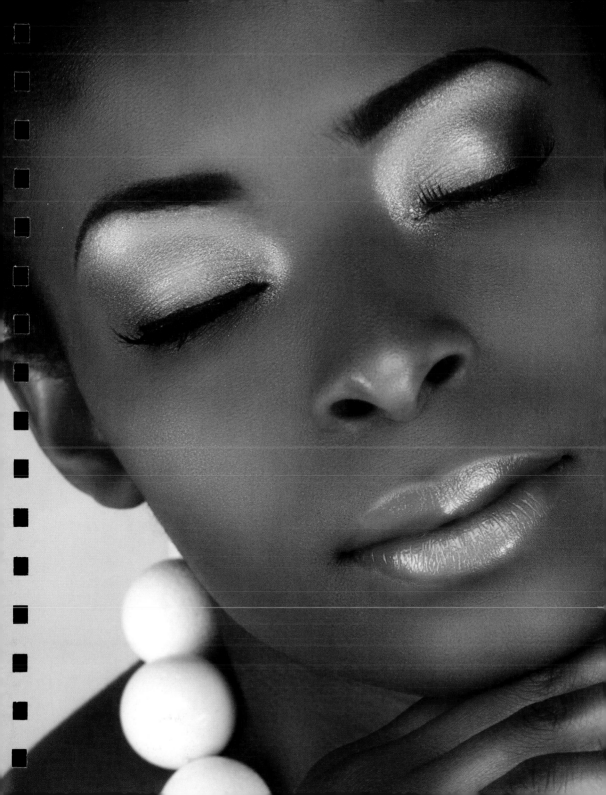

Equipment for eyebrows

Slanted eyebrow brush This brush has a slanted edge, which enables an even application across the brow. It should be held so that the longer end is closer to the eye and it follows the shorter end. The brush is thin and is made of firm fibers. It should be used with eyebrow powder.

Eyebrow powder This powder is matte and comes in a range of colors to match all hair colors. It is used to fill and/or reshape the eyebrows.

Eyebrow wand This is the same shape as a mascara wand. It can be used to brush through the eyebrows to groom them.

Tweezers To pluck eyebrows into a shape and groom stray hairs, invest in a good quality pair of tweezers with slanted ends that sit together squarely when closed. Poor quality tweezers will make plucking very painful. Grab the hair as close to the root as possible, first close the tweezers on the hair and pull gently to check you haven't caught any skin, and then pull them away firmly and quickly in the direction of growth.

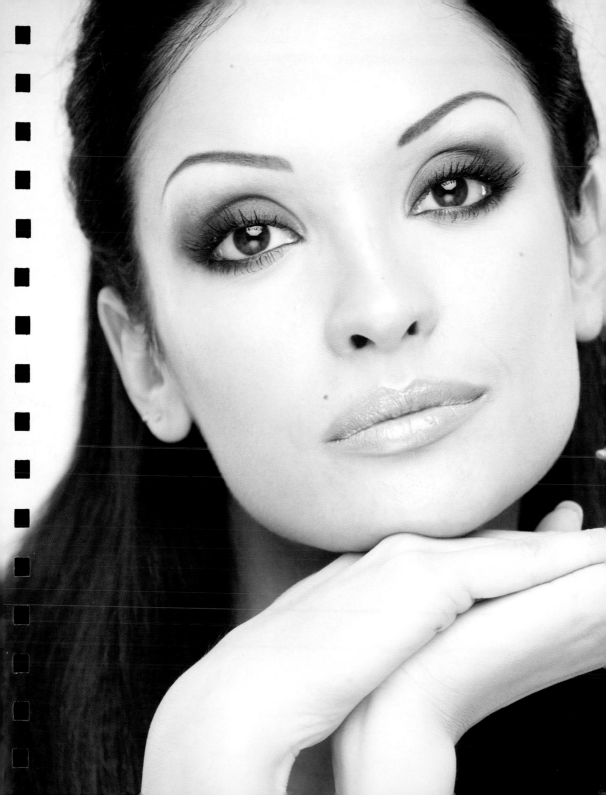

Eyebrow shaping

→ step 1

First comb through your eyebrows to remove any powder or foundation and to get all the hairs lying in the same direction.

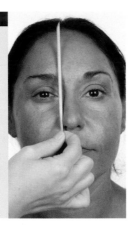

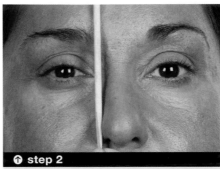

↑ step 2

To locate where the brow should start, hold an orange stick, or something straight and thin, vertically against the face. The stick should connect the side of the bridge of the nose, the inner corner of the eye, and the starting point for the eyebrow. The side of the bridge of the nose is a better marker than the edge of the nostril as nose shapes vary.

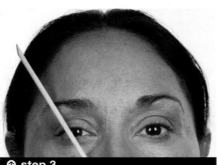

↑ step 3

To locate the correct place for the arch of the brow, look straight ahead and join the bottom of the bridge of the nose with the outer edge of the pupil. The place where the stick crosses the brow gives you the ideal place for the arch. To locate the finish point for the eyebrow, join the bottom of the bridge of the nose with the outer corner of the eye—where the stick hits the browbone is where the eyebrow should end.

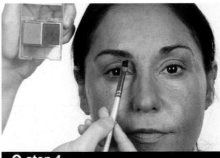

↑ step 4

Having located and marked these places, fill the brow with pencil or powder in a shade similar to the color of the natural eyebrow hairs.

Eyebrow shapes and solutions

We have hair above our eyes to keep moisture out of our eyes. The natural arch channels water and sweat around the side of the eyes. Styling eyebrows dates back to the Egyptians, and through the ages various styles and shapes have been in fashion. Today the fashion is for more naturally groomed eyebrows, but in the 1950s it was fashionable to have heavy, thick brows. When styling eyebrows, it is easy to get it wrong; page 114 describes some common eyebrow mistakes many women make.

Perfect shape

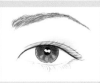

Consult an eyebrow professional initially for help in determining your best eyebrow shape. It's well worth the time and money. Once you've had the initial shaping done professionally, you can maintain it easily at home. The shape follows the line of the eye and isn't overplucked. The arch is in the right place and it is soft and subtle.

Overplucked

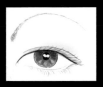

An overplucked brow is very unflattering, making the nose look larger and the eyes seem too far apart. It is also incredibly aging. You can make this mistake when you are trying to create more and more of an arch but aren't sure where it should be. Fill in what is left with a soft color and try to grow all the hairs back before you shape them again.

Straight

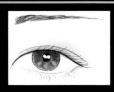

A straight eyebrow is when the arch of the eyebrow never existed or has disappeared from too much tweezing. It is the hardest eyebrow to fix and usually can't be done with pencil or powder. Let the hairs grow back and try to create more of an arched shape.

The triangle

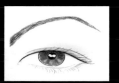

The arch is in the wrong place, usually too far out. This can happen when the angle of hair growth changes sharply at the arch. This shape can make the eyelid look puffy or the eyes look crossed! Fill in the gap under the eyebrow and tweeze a few more hairs so the arch moves inward.

Tadpole or comma

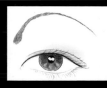

This eyebrow is overplucked and starts with a small ball at the inner corner. It is easy to make this mistake if the hair at the inner corner of the brow grows upward while the rest of the hairs grow outward. To smooth the sharp angle, fill in the gap, filling out the brow and softening the angle.

114 essential techniques

Eyebrow mistakes

Unsymmetrical brows

The two sides of your face are not identical, so it is unlikely both your eyebrows are exactly the same shape. To avoid enhancing this, don't use a small mirror, use one big enough to see your whole face. Pluck your eyebrows simultaneously, matching one to the other. Fill to correct them if necessary.

Eyebrow color clashes with hair color

This can happen if your hair is turning gray but your eyebrows aren't, or if you dye your hair a completely different shade than your natural color. You can darken your brows with pencil or powder or you could consider tinting or bleaching your eyebrows, but get it done professionally.

Tattooed eyebrows

There are two reasons people do this: if brows have been overplucked and have disappeared, or because the natural shape is undesirable. Tattooing looks very harsh and should be avoided. The color is always wrong and it never fades.

Stencils

This looks very fake and has nothing to do with the natural shape. Stencils are often too dark and positioned incorrectly.

Brow tips

- When done correctly, brow powder looks more natural than pencil.
- Work with the natural shape of your brows as much as possible. Let the shape guide you when grooming and shaping.
- To check the desired shape before you remove any hairs, color the ones you are going to remove with a white pencil or concealer.
- Thin eyebrows tend to make your face look instantly older. Don't overdo it.

COMMON PROBLEMS

Most people have something they are not happy with, but applying the right makeup can help us feel better about these little imperfections.

● Under-eye bags

Constant puffiness under the eye, commonly called eye bags, is a hereditary problem. It is caused by the structure of the eye beneath the lower eyelid where the fat, which normally lies beneath the eyeball and acts as a shock absorber, is displaced. Eye creams cannot treat this problem. The problem can become more visible as you get older, as the skin naturally thins and becomes less elastic.

Instead of constantly battling with eye bags, some people occasionally wake up with puffy eyes after a late night or a bad night's sleep. If this is the case you can use a cold compress to decrease them. Soak two cotton pads in cold milk and rest against closed eyes for 10 minutes.

To use makeup to counteract puffiness under the eye, shade the area that sticks out using a concealer or foundation one or two shades darker than the skin tone, to make it appear flatter. The color choice depends on how much puffiness there is. Try the light shade first and if it doesn't achieve the desired effect, darken it further.

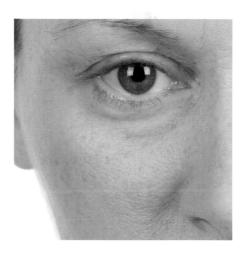

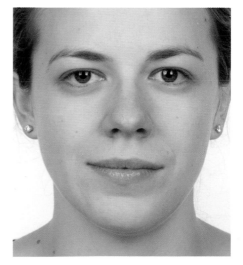

❍ Uneven lips

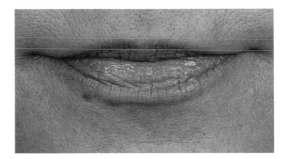

If your lips are visibly unsymmetrical, you can use lipliner to balance the shape. Match the thinner side to the fuller side, drawing outside of the lip line. Make sure your pencil is freshly sharpened for a precise application of the liner and draw with a very steady hand. Always use a natural-colored lipliner. I would advise sticking to natural shades of lipstick and gloss. If the results look unnatural, apply a natural lip color to your lips and use natural or clear gloss. The gloss will blur the edges of the lip and make the unevenness less visible. Finally, draw attention away from your lips by making a statement with your eyes.

❍ Oily T-zone

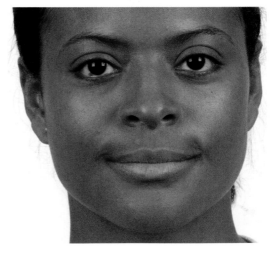

It is very common to be shiny across the forehead and down the center of the nose. This does not mean you have oily skin. You can't stop your skin from producing oils; it is a natural process. To minimize shine try using a matte primer. This will keep the oils at bay for longer. Instead of piling on loads of dense powder, which will eventually become cakey, use a loose translucent powder or a pressed blotting powder. Both will control shine without adding lots of product. Between powder applications, use oil blotting papers; press against the skin, hold for a couple of seconds, remove, and move to the next area.

◑ Bumpy skin

Problems with skin texture cannot be fixed overnight. Implement a good skin care routine, however, and you will see results in the long-term. Regularly exfoliate the skin and use face masks. In the short-term, use a makeup primer to even out skin tone and smooth the surface. Feel the consistency of primers before choosing one—a thicker consistency will work best. Avoid blushers, bronzers, or highlighters that contain shimmer.

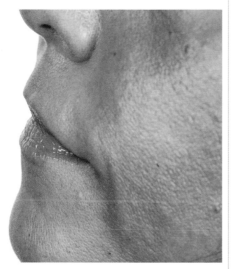

◑ Blemishes/Acne

If you never suffer from blemishes, you are very lucky and in a minority! To conceal a blemish, you should not use the same shade or consistency of concealer used under the eyes. The area under the eye is generally lightened, and using this shade on a blemish will highlight it rather than concealing it!

When blemishes are raised lumps under the skin, apply a suitable concealer that matches your skin tone (nothing too creamy) over the raised area with a concealer brush, starting at the center and blending outward until it disappears into the surrounding skin. If it still appears raised, apply a concealer one shade

darker than your skin tone directly onto the raised area. To get a precise application, use a small concealer brush and gently pat with the pad of your index finger to blend. Using a velour puff, press loose powder over the top to set; pressing the puff lightly onto the skin and then removing it, ensuring you don't drag or disturb the product.

If you have squeezed or picked a blemish and it is weeping, it will be very hard to get concealer to stick to it and also the concealer will go into the open pore and cause further irritation, so you should avoid using it until there is a scab. Once a scab has formed you can apply concealer on it. First apply concealer over the whole area with a concealer brush, blending the edges. When you have applied the concealer the edges of the scab or any raised or sunken areas will be visible. You may need to go over the edge with a small concealer brush to get a smooth finish and also apply lighter or darker concealer to any sunken or raised areas. If the blemish has dried out or if the skin is flaky, you may find a liquid or cream concealer easier to apply. It conceals better than one with a waxier consistency.

If you suffer from acne, there are two things to avoid. The first is using a heavy base all over your face. The second is using a light base all over your face and having to pile on concealer. It is better to use a liquid base with light to medium coverage all over your face, wait for it to settle, and then apply a

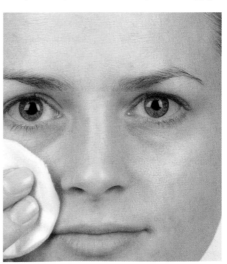

second layer over the parts of the face that are affected with acne. Once the second layer has settled, you can assess how much additional coverage you require from concealer. If the acne has a lot of redness in it, use a green tinted primer to even the tone. If you don't have a concealer brush, use a cotton swab.

Dehydrated skin

Dry and dehydrated skin are not the same thing (see page 26 for the common causes of dry skin). Dry skin is deficient in natural oils; dehydrated skin is lacking water. If you strip natural oils and moisture from your skin, you are making it harder for your skin to do what it is meant to do naturally.

To combat dehydrated skin:
- drink lots of water
- use an oil-based cleanser
- avoid products containing alcohol
- don't regularly use makeup wipes
- Always use moisturizer in the morning and at night use a heavier night cream or a combination of moisturizer and serum.

Makeup and dehydrated skin:
- Before applying makeup, apply moisturizer and wait a few minutes for it to sink into the skin.
- Use a moisturizing foundation and especially avoid oil-free products.
- Use cream blush instead of a powder.

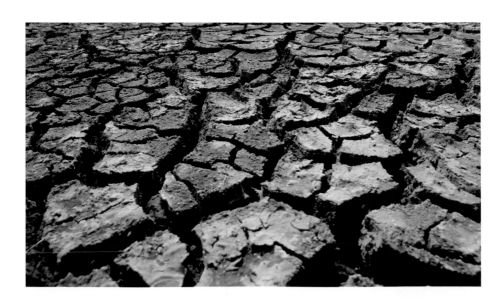

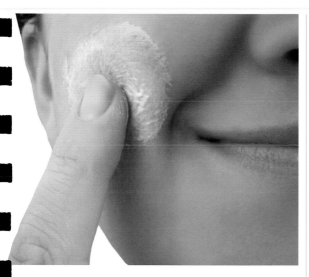

● Sun-damaged skin

Always use SPF coverage when you are outside, whether it is summer or winter. You can get protection from a moisturizer or foundation that has an SPF, or you can double up and use both. Your skin's memory is longer than your own—it will never forget sun damage, making areas weak that have once been damaged so they are prone to repeated burning. Prolonged unprotected sun exposure causes premature aging and sunspots. To add natural warmth to your skin, use makeup or a moisturizer that builds a gradual fake tan.

● Dry flaky skin

Use a rich moisturizer day and night. In the morning let it settle into your skin and then use a moisturizing foundation. If you have a shiny T-zone, dust lightly with translucent powder but don't use it with a heavy hand and don't apply with a powder puff, as the product will collect around the flaky skin. Use a cream blush instead of powder.

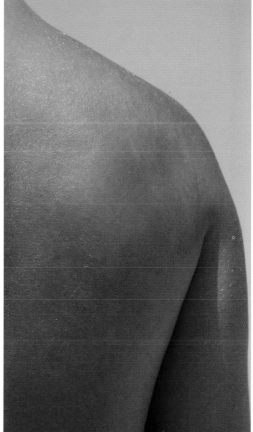

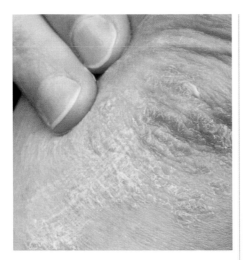

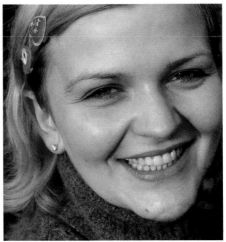

⬆ Eczema

There are millions of eczema sufferers around the world. Eczema is an allergic condition that affects the skin. It is a form of dermatitis. It can vary in degrees of severity from moderate to severe. You should consult your doctor, naturopath, or dermatologist for advice and treatment creams.

Avoid perfumed soaps, shampoos, and moisturizers. Look for products that have anti-inflammatory and emollient ingredients, and avoid anything that contains lanolin. Use organic and mineral makeup that has few ingredients and is hypoallergenic and natural.

Eyelids are commonly affected. Use powder eyeshadows with a matte finish, as shimmer particles can cause irritation. Mascara and eye makeup should be water-soluble so there is no need to use harsh eye makeup removers.

Sweating

It is very common to sweat. Some people sweat more easily than others, but at some stage we all experience it. If your face gets sweaty, blot it with a tissue. Don't rub as this will disturb your makeup. You can carry a small travel spray bottle containing water and spritz your face to cool it down; this will also freshen your makeup. Try to increase the air flow around your face, as the extra air will evaporate the water on the surface.

⬆ Scars/Birthmarks

There are special concealers available to cover scars, birthmarks, and even tattoos (these are referred to as camouflage makeup). Depending on the depth of color you are covering, several layers can be required. You should build up the cover one layer at a time, using a concealer brush. If you use your fingers, you will move the product away from the area you are trying to cover. When you have covered the area sufficiently, set it with loose powder to stop the makeup from transferring onto clothes. Press the powder with a velour puff, ensuring you don't drag the puff against the skin and disturb the product. If you are covering a scar that has a red undertone, first apply a green color corrector, then a thin layer of foundation. Then begin to layer on camouflage makeup until the scar is no longer visible.

Facial hair

Facial hair can either be inherited or caused by a hormone imbalance. There are currently three ways to have unwanted hair removed: electrolysis, waxing, and laser treatment. Waxing is not a long-term solution. Electrolysis is a permanent solution but requires a course of treatments. Laser hair removal is permanent and immediate but may require additional treatments. Some women choose not to remove hair and bleach it instead.

Makeup can sit on top of facial hair or collect around it, so don't go for a heavy application, especially of powder.

◓ Fine Lines/Wrinkles

As we get older, fine lines and wrinkles become more apparent. The key to keeping them at bay for as long as possible is hydrating the skin with moisturizers, encouraging cell turnover by exfoliating regularly, and using an eye cream.

Use creamy foundation that won't collect in any creases and a lip primer or pencil to create a barrier at the edge of your lips and stop lipstick bleeding. To minimize the appearance of fine lines and wrinkles, apply a highlighter or pale concealer directly onto the deepest part, using a small concealer brush, after applying foundation.

Lightly smudge with your finger to blend.Plumping creams are available; they temporarily reduce the depth of fine lines and wrinkles by encouraging more blood to flow close to the surface of the skin. A plumping cream should be applied to totally clean skin before moisturizer and makeup are used.

Heterochromia

It is not uncommon to have subtly different eye colors. Some people choose to wear colored contact lenses, but here are some tips for rebalancing the eye colors with makeup:

- Use eye colors from the same color family, applied to each eye with varying levels of shading to create a balanced effect.
- Draw the attention away from the color of your eyes by using bright colors on the lids.
- A smoky eye look is great for framing the eye and drawing the attention away from the eye itself.

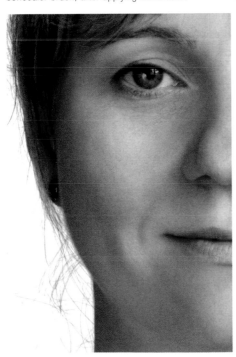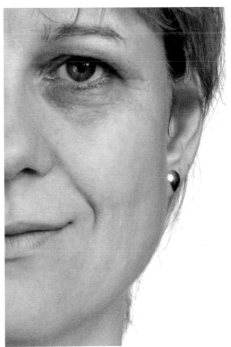

AGING

Every woman is different and the decade in which the skin blossoms will vary. No matter what your age, for great skin you should drink lots of water, stay out of the sun, and avoid cigarette smoke.

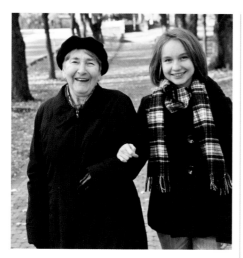

Changing faces

In your twenties, you may have beautifully clear, glowing skin not tarnished by age, but some women may still be suffering from teenage acne. Your skin cells regenerate fast, so your complexion should be even and radiant—there is no need for a heavy base, just a great concealer for blemishes. In your thirties you need to be preventing future problems. Start using eye cream and a good moisturizer, and develop a more sophisticated makeup look. Start to include regular exfoliation in your skin care routine to maintain radiance as cell turnover begins to slow. In your forties your skin can become drier and feel looser. This can

lead to wrinkles, so use a serum under your moisturizer for lift, and a night cream for hydration. Use a primer under foundation to fill in fine lines and wrinkles.

Teens

In your teens major changes occur hormonally that affect your skin. Teenagers are commonly plagued by acne and blemishes and are constantly at war with their skin. Even if you are one of the unlucky ones,

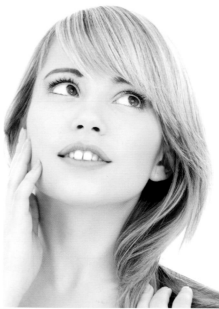

don't wear too heavy a foundation. You are piling on the years if your makeup is too dense. Use a light foundation, layering to build up the coverage, and use concealer where necessary. If you have problem skin, get advice on how best to treat it and follow a skin care regime. Look at fashion magazines for makeup inspiration, play with colors, and experiment.

20s

This should be the best time for you and your skin. It is naturally radiant and full of elasticity; the signs of aging have not yet appeared; and the problems of teenage skin are behind you.

You don't need a complicated skin care regime as long as you have some sort of regime in place. Don't forget to moisturize your neck, hands, and around your eyes. Get into good habits and always remove your makeup at the end of the day. Whatever the current trend is, do not overpluck your eyebrows. The hair here thins as you age and overplucking now will mean no eyebrows at all by the time you're forty! If you are still suffering from blemishes, use oil-free products and regularly steam your face to open pores and flush them out. Celebrate the radiance of your skin and let it show through your makeup. Don't go for anything too heavy. Use a concealer where you need extra cover and be as bold as you want with makeup, but take the time to perfect how you apply it so it has a more sophisticated finish.

30s

The production of sebum and cell turnover have both begun to slow, so the first signs of aging may make themselves known as a few lines and drier skin. Do everything you can to slow down the process. Wear sunscreen every day—a good way of doing this with minimum hassle or expense is to buy a moisturizer with SPF. Drink lots of water, exercise, and establish healthy eating habits. Respect your skin. A good daily regime is essential and weekly exfoliation is highly recommended. Use face masks and, if you are able to, go for facials. For years to come, you will get out

what you put in. Use an eye cream at least once daily. There is no excuse not to remove your makeup at the end of the day. Annoyingly, although you are beginning to feel and see the effects of aging, blemishes are still about. Blemishes at this age should not be treated with the products aimed at younger

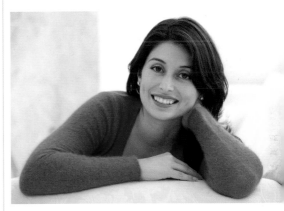

skins, which are oilier—they are too drying on a slightly older skin. In your thirties you become more sure of who you are and so you're under less pressure to always be at the height of fashion. As with clothes, decide what suits you and what doesn't and learn the techniques required to achieve these looks with a professional finish. Instead of taking inspiration from the runway, take it from the red carpet. Makeup on the red carpet follows trends, but it is more sophisticated. Runway makeup is too bold, and replicating it should be left to teenagers and those in their twenties. Your makeup should be sophisticated and sexy. You may have less time on your hands if juggling a career and a family, so use products that double up, such as cream blushes that can also be used on the lips and even on the eyes.

40s

In your forties it is hard not to feel the pressure of aging. Fine lines you had toward the end of your thirties deepen as you approach fifty. Enjoy the fact you are comfortable in your own skin, and with the right skin care regime you can continue to look

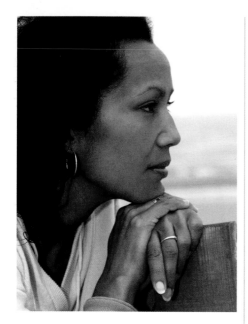

fresher and brighter it makes you feel and other people will notice and comment on the change. There is no harm in getting a makeup lesson to learn the correct techniques.

Start to fill in your eyebrows. They may be naturally thinning, and well-groomed brows are very sophisticated and frame the eyes as well as drawing attention to the whole eye and away from any lines.

50s and beyond

Cell turnover is almost half what it was when you were younger, so your complexion can look dull. Wrinkles and fine lines are visible as skin loses collagen, beause skin is thinner, and after menopause also drier. Use moisturizers that boost collagen. Use cream cleanser, as wetting and drying the skin promotes dryness. Avoid alcohol-based toners. Use eye cream that is specifically formulated for more mature skin. Even if you feel you can't reverse what has already happened or have not before had a good skin care regime, it's never too late to start to slow down what is going to happen in the future.

Primer comes into its own now to smooth the texture of the skin, making makeup easier to apply and giving a smoother, longer-lasting finish. An illuminator can give the skin a youthful radiance, and a moisturizing foundation such as a cream foundation works best. Foundation will even skin tone. If you have broken capillaries or rosacea, use a green-tinted primer or lightly dust bronzer on top of foundation as this counteracts redness.

As eyebrows and eyelashes thin with age, add definition to your eyebrows and around the eyes. Powders look more natural and are easy to use. Use blush to lift the complexion and add a youthful glow. Use warm, rich eye colors, and make sure you work the products into the eyes in all directions because the looser skin can crease so parts of the eyelid are easily missed.

youthful. The skin care and moisturizer you used in your twenties will not be suitable now. Shop around and be open to new brands and creams. Your skin gets drier with age, as it is not able to retain moisture as well as it did when you were younger. Use a rich moisturizer and a serum at night, as well as eye cream and a lighter cream moisturizer, instead of lotion, in the day. Regularly exfoliate and use masks. Masks will help to keep the skin looking radiant. Drink lots of water and make sure your diet includes antioxidants such as fresh fruit and vegetables. Choose makeup colors and looks that suit your age. Making yourself feel younger by piling on heavy makeup in inappropriate colors will not make you look younger. There is no reason not to update your makeup with a version of what is currently in fashion, but tone down the looks and colors to make them appropriate to what suits you. You need to wear more makeup than you did in your teens and twenties (although not every teenager realizes this!), but it needs to be the right makeup, applied correctly. Take a fresh look at your face. If you have always worn blushes in the same tone, try a new color. You will be amazed at how much

Summer vs. Winter

	Summer	Winter
Foundation	Warmer weather and sunshine naturally even skin tone, so use a lighter formula or mix foundation with moisturizer to make it more sheer. You can switch to an oil-free formula in the summer if you get shiny quickly in warm weather.	To combat dryness use a creamy formula in winter and always use moisturizer underneath.
Blusher	A powder blush will help control shine by absorbing excess oils. A bronzer will warm up the skin and is a sensible alternative to having your face in the sun. Peach-toned blush is flattering on bronzed skin.	Cream-based blush is hydrating and will keep your skin moisturized for longer, especially if you are going to be outside for a prolonged period.
Lipstick/gloss	Matte lipsticks and stains are good for adding natural color that lasts. Glosses can melt in very hot weather and slide straight off. Look for products that have built-in sunscreen.	Tinted lips balms are a good option as they provide hydration as well as color. Choose lipstick in a moisture-rich formula. Lip gloss stays put for longer in winter.
Mascara	Waterproof mascara is a good choice for vacations or if you find your normal mascara smudges in hot weather. If it still smudges, curl your lashes and use clear mascara. If you have fair lashes, consider having them tinted.	You can use waterproof or normal mascara in winter.
Eyeshadow	Cream eyeshadows have a tendency to crease anyway but will do so even more in warm weather. Apply foundation over the eyelid and press in loose powder to set. This will control the oils and keep your eyeshadow crease-free for longer. If it does crease, use your finger to work the product back out of the creases and dust with loose powder to set again.	Use an eye cream to stop the thinner skin around your eyes becoming dry.

Chapter 3

DEVELOPING LOOKS

Now that you have mastered the basic essential
techniques, it is time to learn how to develop these
into different looks to suit your mood or the occasion.
Using the basic scale on the following pages will
enable you to see how to vary the intensity of a
particular look to make it appropriate for different
styles, tastes, and situations.

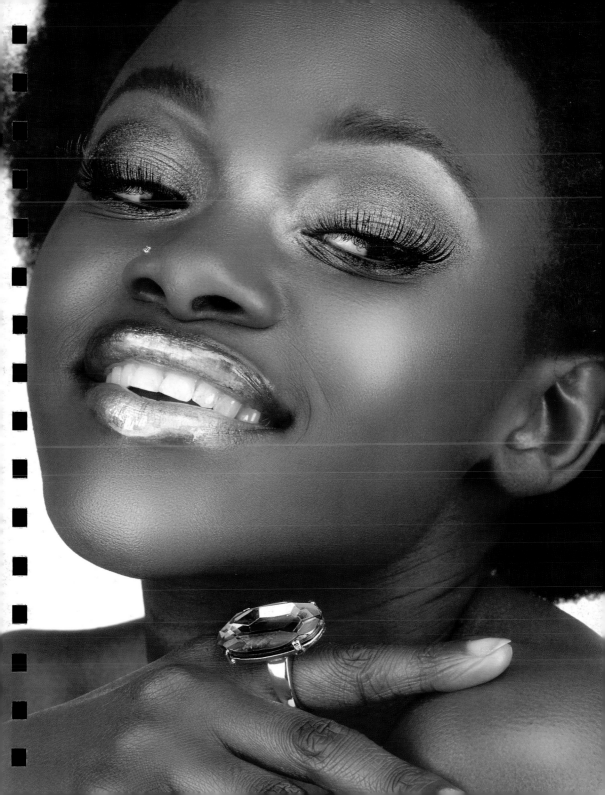

PLANNING A MAKEUP LOOK

Whether you are entertaining at home or going for a job interview, it is good for your self-esteem if you make an effort to look your best. More than one makeup look is needed to suit the various roles you find yourself playing from day to day.

You have your basic everyday makeup look. The makeup you would do for daytime may vary from workday to weekend, but the looks are ones you use over and over, maybe just changing an eye color or lip color to suit the season or the clothes you are wearing. When it comes to a night out or special occasion, you should give a little more thought to what makeup look you are going to do.

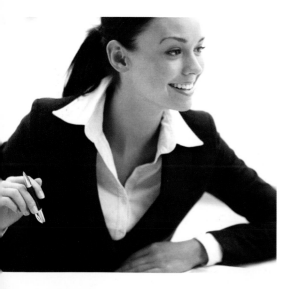

This will always be met with positive comments from those around you and will stop you from getting into a makeup rut and looking the same all the time.

Before an event, you always think about what you are going to wear, whether you need to buy something new, or take your outfit to the dry cleaners, as well as which shoes and accessories you will wear. You should also include in this planning what makeup look would suit the outfit, occasion, and you. Do you have the products needed to achieve the makeup look or do you need to purchase additional products?

When I am doing someone's makeup for a special event, I will always start with a consultation, asking lots of questions to build up a picture in my head of what makeup I am going to do. These questions are ones you can take into account yourself when planning makeup for a special occasion.

These are the questions I ask:

- What is the event/occasion?
- What time of day does it start and finish?
- What color are you going to wear?
- What is the style of your outfit?
- How will you style your hair?
- What colors are you comfortable wearing?
- Have your seen any pictures of makeup that inspire you?

Ask yourself all these questions and then consider the following:

Makeup inspiration and choice should be taken from the color of the clothes you are going to wear. Your makeup shouldn't clash with any bold colors, and you should choose complimentary colors from the same color palette. If you are going to wear all black with neutral accessories, definitely introduce color or a wow factor with the makeup.

Is there a period feel to your outfit choice? Does it lean toward one era more than any other? You may also choose to go for a hairstyle and makeup that lean toward the same period. It is usually best to do this with a modern twist.

If the start time is during the day—a wedding for example—don't go for a heavy look as it may be too much in daylight. Instead, tone down the look for the daytime part of the event but have a touch-up kit in your handbag so you can add more intensity once day turns to night.

If you are really unsure about color choice, stick to browns or grays. These go with everything and you can work on the scale of intensity, making the makeup more glamorous than you would for daytime.

Before you start applying your makeup, consider your plan, even if it's just in your head. If you are doing a smoky eye, do the eyes first so you can clear up any fallen product. Be realistic about how long it is going to take you and allow enough time to do a good job.

Don't stress yourself out on the day of an important event. If you have planned your look in advance and it involves something you are not 100% confident about, such as a strong red lip or false eyelashes, practice beforehand.

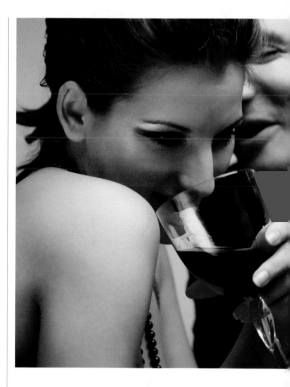

Pro Tip

Before you start applying your makeup, lay out all the products and tools you are going to use so that everything is on hand. Select a few key items to take with you for touch-ups, and don't forget brushes or a puff if required.

EVERYDAY MAKEUP

It's all about the eyes. You can vary the intensity of a look by altering the shade and intensity of the eye color you are using. For a basic look where only the intensity is altered, use natural browns or grays. This same look can be achieved using other colors.

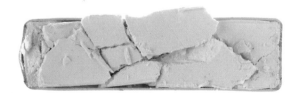

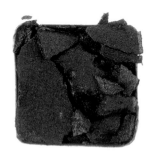
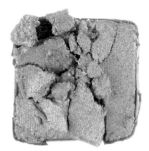
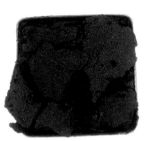

Light

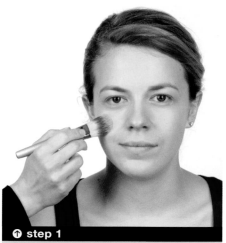

↑ step 1

After priming the face, apply foundation all over, including the eyelids. Start in the center and blend outward toward the hairline and jawline. See page 46.

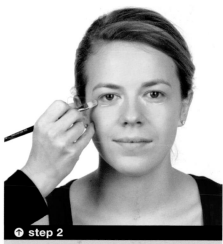

↑ step 2

Using a mirror, assess where you need more cover. Apply concealer as required around the eyes, nose, and mouth, and over any redness or blemishes. See page 50.

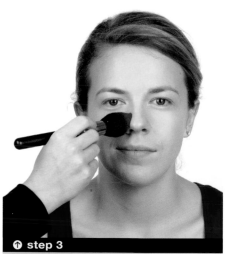

↑ step 3

Set the foundation and concealer by applying powder. Focus on the T-zone and lightly dust over the rest of the face, including the eyes. See page 56.

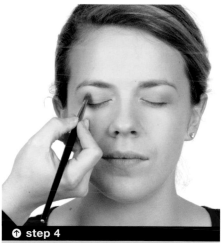

↑ step 4

As a base, apply nude matte shadow all over the eyelids from the lash line to the brow. This will help with blending and evening the tone of the eyelid. Lighten under the arch of the brow and inner corner of the eye using a paler eyeshadow to open the eye; apply soft gray shadow from the lash line to the socket.

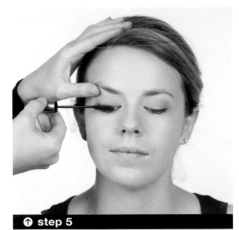

↑ step 5

Curl the eyelashes and apply one coat of mascara to the top lashes.

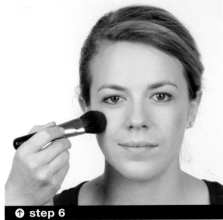

↑ step 6

For a healthy fresh glow, apply bronzer to the high points of the face, where the sun would naturally tan the skin, and use a fresh pink blusher on the apple of the cheeks.

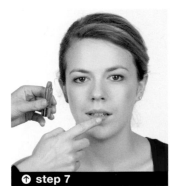

↑ step 7

Stain lips by lightly pressing a warm pink lipstick into the center of the lips with your finger. Blot to remove any oils and then add clear gloss on top.

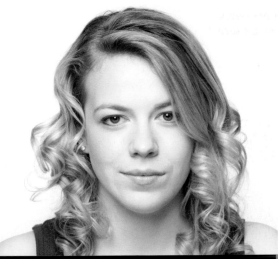

Pro tip

If you want more definition around the eyes, softly line along the top and bottom lashes with a stronger gray powder eyeshadow close to the root of the lashes. See page 98.

Variations on a light look

How to vary a light makeup look to suit your age, skin tone, eye shape, and the season.

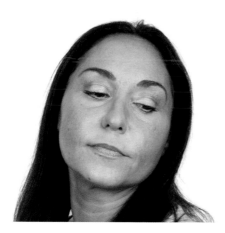

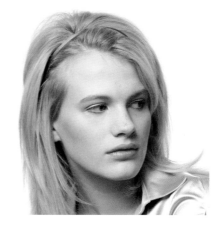

For a light look on darker skin, use shades from the brown scale, from beige to mid-brown. Matte colors or those with a slight sheen work better on older faces.

For a fresh, summery look on a younger face, use color. This is still a light daytime look, as the color is applied as a wash and darkened only along the lashes, not in the socket.

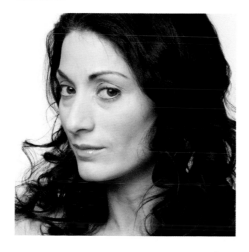

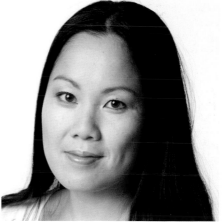

Subtle bronze and gold are a good choice for Mediterranean or tanned skin, as they will flatter the complexion. Complement with glowing peachy or apricot blush, and natural glossy lips.

For a light makeup look on Asian eyes, define along the lash line with eyeliner and use subtle colors such as pink, complemented with gold on the eyelids. Take the color above the crease and blend the edges well. Use a soft color on the lips.

Medium

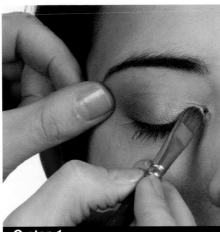

⬆ step 1

After applying foundation, concealer, and powder (see pages 46, 50, and 56), apply nude matte eyeshadow all over the eyelids from the lash line to the brow as a base for your eye makeup. This will help with blending and evening out the tone of the eyelid. Lighten under the arch of the brow and inner corner of the eye with a paler eyeshadow to open the eye.

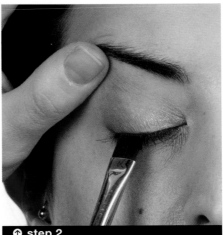

⬆ step 2

Line along the top lashes with a matte dark brown powder, using a fine detail or flat liner brush. Pull your eyelid taut so the line is solid. The skin on your eyelid is loose and can ruffle up slightly, which can give a broken eye line. First work along the lashes from the outer corner inward. If you have crepey eyelids, go back over the line outward.

➔ step 3

Add a small amount of champagne shimmer on the high point in the center of the eyelid. If your skin tone is darker, go for a mid-color shimmer eyeshadow.

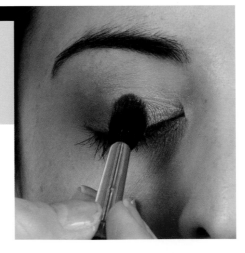

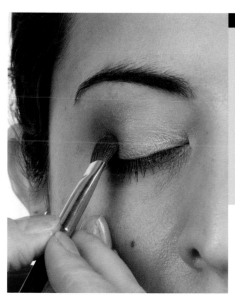

⊖ step 4

Enhance the outer third of the eyelid with a mid-brown eyeshadow, blended in from the lash line up to the socket. Blend inward along the socket line, slightly following the natural curved shape of the eye. Build the color up a little at a time until you are satisfied with the intensity. If you have a darker skin tone, adjust the color of the eyeshadow so it is darker than your skin tone.

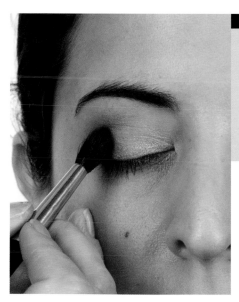

⊖ step 5

Blend together to soften the edges, using a clean blending brush. Add definition along the bottom lash line by applying the mid-brown eyeshadow close to the root of the lashes with a detail brush. Curl the lashes and apply one coat of mascara.

Pro Tip

The skill professionals have that sets them apart is the ability to blend makeup so that everything seamlessly blends together. For eyes, use a clean blending brush (or the one you use for nude/pale colors) and soften around the edges and the seam between colors so they merge and fade into one another.

step 6

Apply blusher and lips to suit your face shape and skin tone. See pages 72 and 80.

Variations on a medium look

Using the same technique and eyeshadow placement, you can adjust the look to suit your age, confidence, and skin tone. Experiment with different colors.

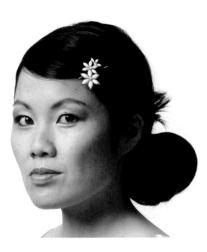

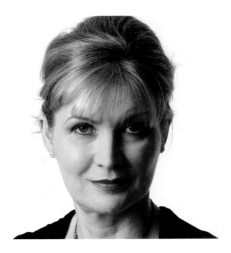

Switch the brown scale colors used in the steps for two colors that complement each other and flatter your skin tone. Here the coral and gold work well together and neither color is too bold.

To vary a medium look and play up another feature, the eyes are made up but are kept light and the lip color is stronger. This works well if you want to make a feature of your lips or draw focus from the eyes.

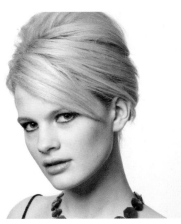

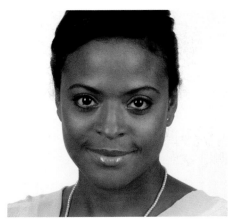

For a polished medium look that is suitable for evening, build the intensity of the eye look by using medium colors that are matte instead of iridescent or shimmery. Play down the other features.

On darker skin tones, adjust the scale of colors so they are darker than the skin tone. Stronger colors are needed when working from the brown or gray scale to make the same impact that you would be able to make with bright colors.

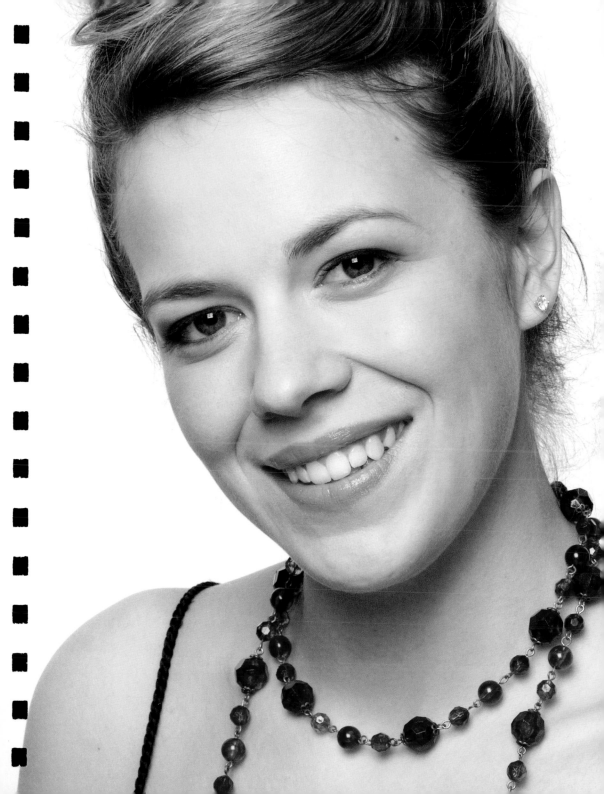

Strong

The smoky brown colors used here could be swapped for grays or bright colors. The principles of applying different colors are the same.

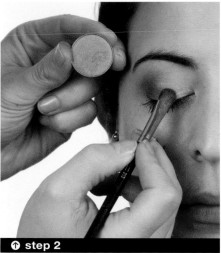

↑ step 2

Apply mid-brown eyeshadow on the outer third of the eyelid and from the lash line up to the socket. Blend inward along the socket line, slightly, following the natural curved shape of the eye. Build the color up a little at a time until you are satisfied with the intensity. If you have a darker skin tone, adjust the color of the eyeshadow so it is darker than your own skin tone.

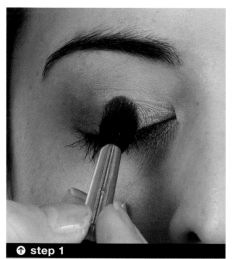

↑ step 1

Follow steps 1, 2, and 3 from page 134.

→ step 3

Build up the intensity of color on the outer part of the eyelid by blending black or dark brown on the outer edge and smudging inward. Take the color above the crease slightly. With your eyes open, mark on the upper part of your eye just above the point that your open eyelid masks, and take the color up to and just above this mark.

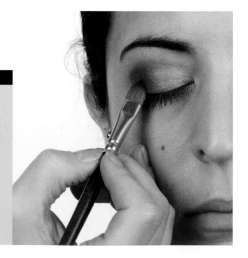

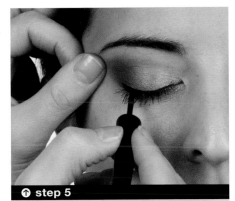

↑ step 4

Apply dark brown or black eyeshadow along the bottom lash line, close to the root of the lashes, using a fine detail brush. This increases the intensity of the look and defines the eye. Brush the powder from the outer corner inward, making short strokes.

↑ step 5

Line along the top lashes with liquid eyeliner. Pull your eyelid taut so the line is solid (the skin on your eyelid is loose and can ruffle up slightly, which can give a broken eye line). Work along the lashes in small strokes, applying from the outer corner inward (see pages 98–100).

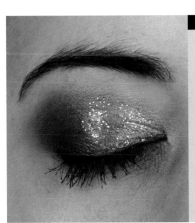

← step 6

Blend the colors on the eye well so there are no hard edges and all the colors melt into each other. To enhance the look further, add gold shimmer or glitter, blending from the inner corner toward the darker shadow. If you are using glitter, use a product that is suspended in water or gel that dries in place; keep your eye closed until it is completely dry. Press it in on top of the eyeshadow so that you don't disturb it. To finish, curl the lashes and apply mascara to the top and bottom lashes. For more intensity use a black kohl pencil along the rim of the lower eyelid.

Pro Tip

When you are doing a strong eye look and using dark or strong colors, do your eye makeup before applying base, concealer, and powder to your face. You can then clear up any fallen product easily and it won't ruin the rest of your makeup (you should still apply foundation over the eye area before doing the makeup).

Variations on a strong look

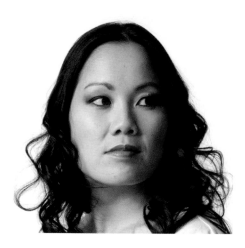

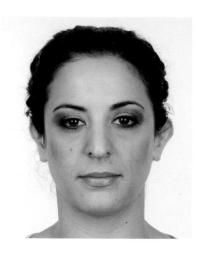

Smoky eyes look great on Asian eyes—just make sure the colors are blended well into each other and the eye area.

For a high-impact evening look, add color. Here I have applied a strong green color all over the eyelid and then added intensity.

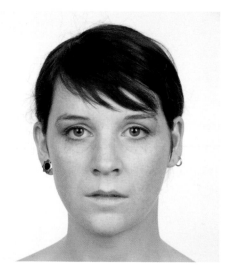

For a strong look on pale skin, use a neutral color over the eyelid and then apply a bold color. Smudge dark brown eyeshadow along the upper and lower lash lines.

➡ You could also try blending black over the outer third of the eyelid, into and above the crease, using black eyeliner along the top lash line.

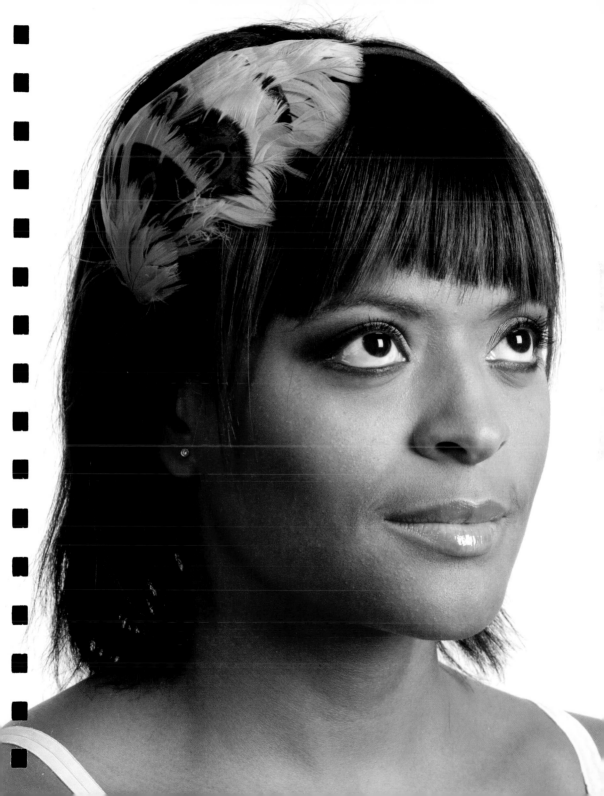

SMOKY EYES

Smoky smoldering eyes take eyeshadow to the next level, creating a look that is sexy and suits different occasions and times of day. Blending and practice are key to perfecting the look.

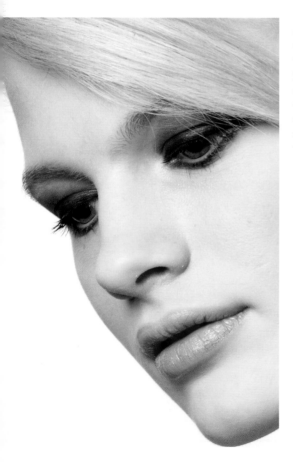

Smoky eyes never go out of fashion and can suit everyone, whatever your age or skin tone. You can vary the intensity of the look depending on the time of day, your wardrobe and style, as well as your age and coloring. You can create smoky eyes using a single color, a couple of tones of the same color, or a contrasting accent color. To make the look stay crease-free all day, layer a cream eye base on after foundation and before using nude matte eyeshadow.

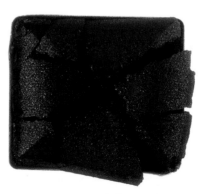

Smoky eyes

For a smoldering sexy look, use matte eyeshadows.

➔ step 1

Do the eyes before applying foundation to your whole face, but do apply foundation over the eyelid first. As a base, brush nude matte shadow all over the eyelids from the lash line to the brow as a base. This will help with blending and evening the tone of the eyelid. Lighten under the arch of the brow and inner corner with a paler eyeshadow to open the eye.

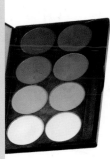
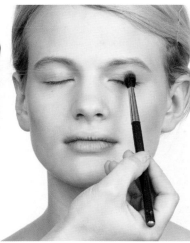

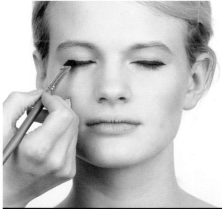

⬆ step 2

Line along the top lashes with black eyeliner. You could use a kohl pencil or (as shown here) a cream eyeliner applied with a flat liner brush (see pages 98–100). Work from the outer corner inward; then to ensure the line is solid, apply from the inner corner outward. The line should be thick and doesn't need to be neat, as it will be smudged and blended over with eyeshadow.

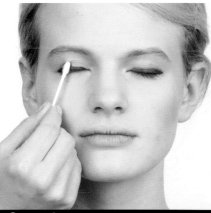

⬆ step 3

Smudge the kohl with a cotton swab. This makes an excellent base for dark eyeshadow and makes the look really intense around the eyes.

➔ step 4

Apply a very dark brown eyeshadow all over the eyelid up to the crease. Layer it on, building up the depth of color. Start on the outer corner of the eye and blend inward. On the outer third, blend the shadow above the crease line. Brush the shadow in all directions so it is a solid application. At this stage, don't worry if the edges are messy—they will be well blended later on.

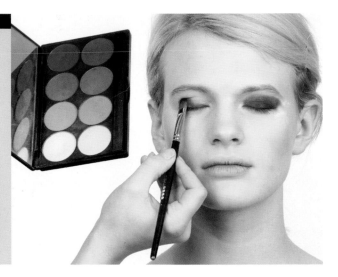

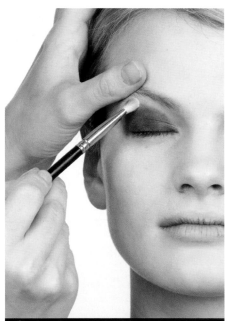

⬆ step 5

To soften the top edge and fade the shadow toward the brow, smudge with a clean brush loaded with nude beige shadow, making small circular movements with your wrist all along the top edge of the dark eyeshadow.

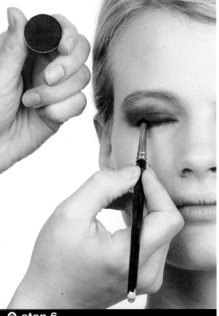

⬆ step 6

Apply a matte black eyeshadow along the lash line with a detail brush, to increase the intensity of the look. Smudge the color downward toward the lash and blend the upper edge into the dark brown.

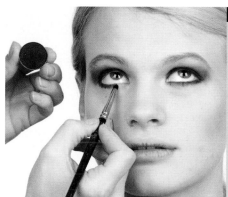

← step 7

Apply matte black eyeshadow along the bottom lash line using a fine detail brush, taking it right up to the root of the lashes, and smudging the color downward. Line the inside rim of the lower eyelid with a black kohl pencil. Curl the eyelashes and apply mascara to the top and bottom eyelashes.

Pro Tip

This look is complemented with subtle contouring blush and nude lips with a touch of gloss.

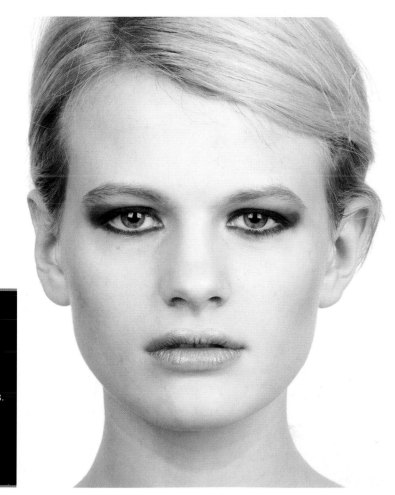

INTRODUCING COLOR

Once you have come to grips with varying the intensity of a look, it is time to experiment with color. Contrary to popular belief, most colors suit most people, if applied properly and blended well. It is important, however, to know what works particularly well for you and your eye color.

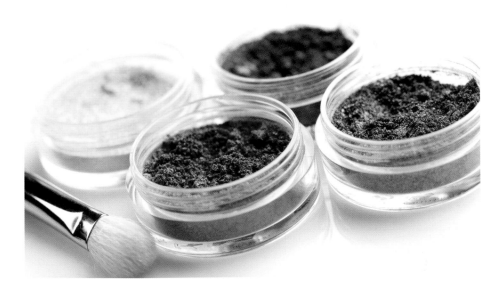

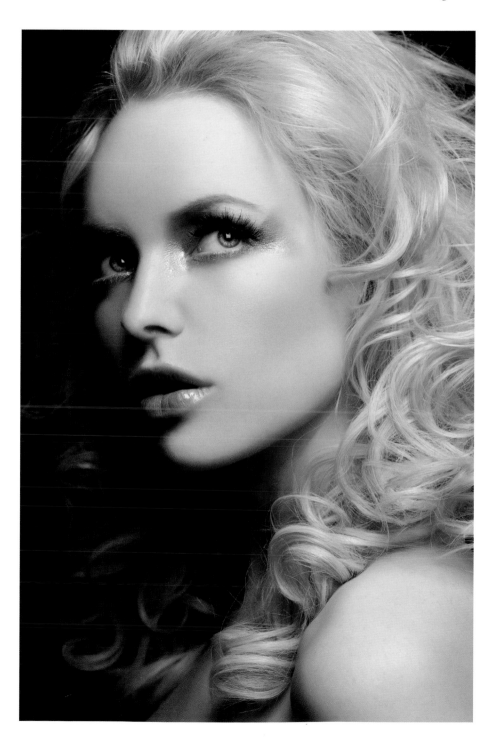

Color theory

It is my belief that anyone can wear any color of makeup as long as they choose the correct shade or hue of color, it is correctly applied, colors used are complementary, and nothing is clashing. Older women can wear color, but it should be more subtle.

To make the right choices when selecting makeup, some understanding of color, how colors are classified, and what colors work together and why, is required. Color is fun and everyone enjoys looking at a color, but it is often very difficult to communicate and accurately describe. For the purpose of makeup, colors are classified in three ways—hue, brightness, and intensity.

- Hue is the difference between pure colors. It is what we are actually asking when we say "what color is that?" If we talk about red, yellow, and blue, what we are describing is the hue.
- Brightness is the range of a color from light to dark. There is a scale of brightness for all colors.
- Intensity is the strength or heaviness of any pure color or point on the gray scale.

Colors used for makeup need to coordinate. The color wheel can help you to understand which colors work together. The common color wheel is an organization of colors in a circle, showing the relationships between the colors considered to be the primary, secondary, and complementary colors.

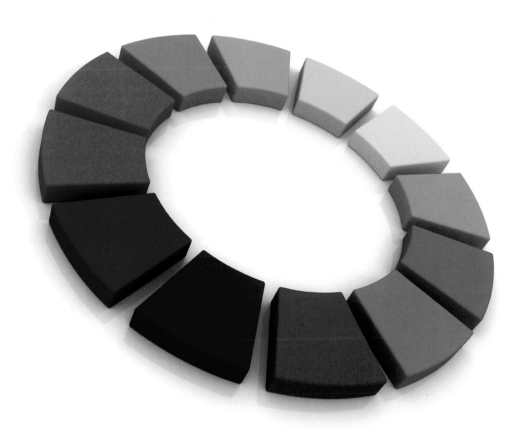

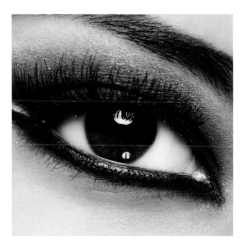

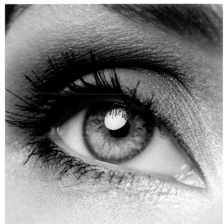

Primary colors in makeup are blue, red, and yellow. Secondary colors are green, orange, and purple. Complementary colors are opposite each other in the color wheel. Colors that complement each other tone each other down; this explains why you use a green-tinted primer if you are prone to redness. If two colors share a pigment, such as blue and green, they are harmonizing colors.

All colors arise from the primary colors. They cannot be made by mixing other colors together. Mixing together equal values of any two primary colors creates the secondary colors.

Use a color wheel to choose colors that work together and to see what shade of a color will work well with your eye, hair, or outfit color, but don't be ruled by it. Experiment with color and if you feel it works for you, go for it!

With makeup it is important to get the tonal difference between colors correct. To make a color into a tint, add white; to create a shade of a color, add black.

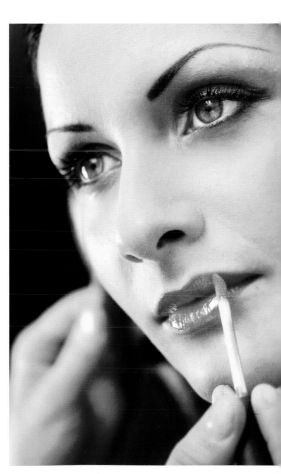

Light brown eyes

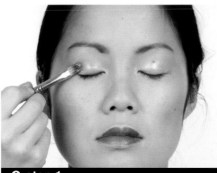

↑ step 1

To prep the eye apply foundation over the eyelid, then brush nude matte shadow all over the eyelid from the lash line to the brow as a base. This will help with blending and evening the tone of the eyelid. To open the eye, lighten under the arch of the brow and inner corner with a paler eyeshadow. Apply a wash of silver eyeshadow over the eyelid up to the crease. Take the color above the crease on the outer third of the eye.

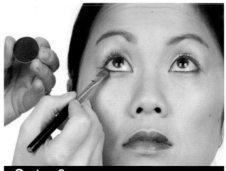

↑ step 2

To frame the eye and define the lash line, apply dark gray or black eyeshadow along the top, close to the root of the lashes (see page 99). Smudge the black into the silver so there isn't a hard edge. Apply the shadow under the bottom lashes close to the roots.

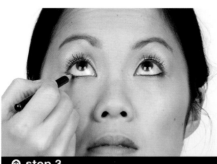

↑ step 3

To increase the intensity of the look, apply black kohl along the inside rim of the lower eyelid. Pull the eyelid taut and apply from the outer corner inward, making short strokes. Curl the lashes and apply mascara (see page 106).

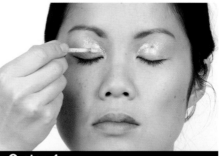

↑ step 4

To add sparkle to this look for a night out or a party, add glitter. It is nice to see the glitter when your eye is open, so apply it over the inner third of the eyelid and above the crease. Use glitter that is suspended in gel or water and press it on so you don't disturb the eyeshadow underneath. Keep your eye closed until it is dry.

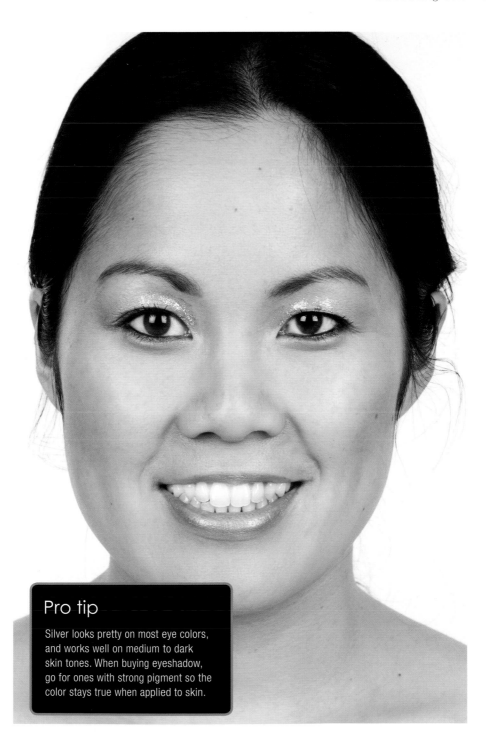

Pro tip

Silver looks pretty on most eye colors, and works well on medium to dark skin tones. When buying eyeshadow, go for ones with strong pigment so the color stays true when applied to skin.

Hazel eyes

⊙ step 1

To prep the eye, apply foundation over the eyelid, then brush nude matte shadow all over from the lash line to the brow to act as a base. This will help with blending and evening the tone of the eyelid. Apply a rich golden shadow over the whole eyelid. With these color tones you often get a richer color from loose pigment. Instead of brushing the product onto the eyelid, press it into your eyelid with your brush. If you are using loose pigment, always do the eyes before applying foundation to the rest of the face as the pigment can fall.

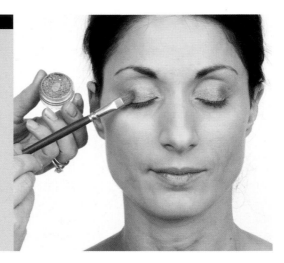

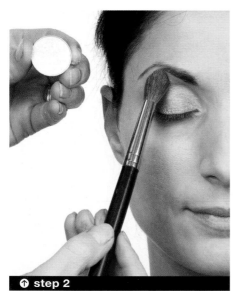

⬆ step 2

Use a matte beige or white powder to highlight under the brow and in the inner corner of the eye. Apply with a blending brush.

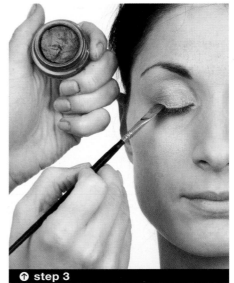

⬆ step 3

Define the lash line with rich dark brown cream liner or eyeshadow. Apply close to the lash line and make sure the line is thin, thickening slightly toward the outer corner. Pull your lid taut when you are drawing the line and start at the outer corner and work inward.

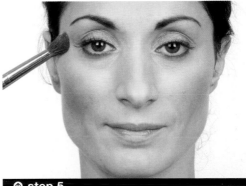

↑ step 4

Line under the bottom lashes right up to the root of the lashes with the same rich brown color, working from the outer corner inward. Fill in the brows if necessary (see page 112), curl the lashes, and apply mascara.

↑ step 5

To complete the golden look, apply bronzer to the highpoints of the face, the cheeks, forehead, nose, and chin. Then apply a warm coral blush. Highlight on top of the cheekbone (see page 60) with a champagne shimmer and apply a coral lip color and touch of gloss.

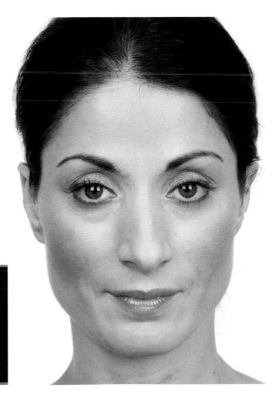

Pro tip

Rich, warm browns, auburns, and gold flatter hazel eyes and a warm skin tone. Browns with a gold shimmer to them are really nice. Cream-to-powder shadows blend well and are long-wearing.

Dark brown eyes

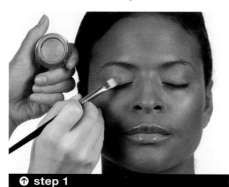

↑ step 1

As an alternative to using foundation as an eye base, apply a cream eyeshadow in a tone similar to the skin. This will neutralize the color of the eyelid, and act as a base for blending other colors and products on top as well as increasing the longevity of the eye makeup.

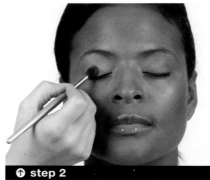

↑ step 2

Because the skin over the eye is very thin, the natural oils in the skin are closer to the surface. To control the oils and prevent the eyeshadow creasing, set the eye base by brushing a matte powder shadow over the top in a similar color. Use a blending brush.

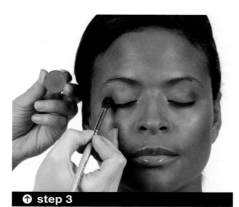

↑ step 3

Enhance the outer third of the eyelid with a mid-brown eyeshadow from the lash line up to the socket. Blend inward along the socket line slightly, following the natural curved shape of the eye. Build the color up a little at a time, until you are satisfied with the intensity. If you have a lighter skin tone, adjust the color of the eyeshadow accordingly.

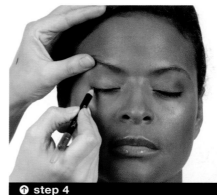

↑ step 4

Line along the top lashes using black eyeliner either from a pot with a flat liner brush or with a pencil. Pull your eyelid taut so the line is solid. The skin on your eyelid is loose and can ruffle up slightly, which can give a broken eye line. Work the liner along the lashes in an outward direction.

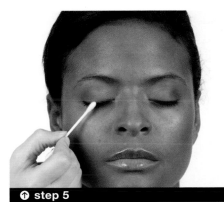

↑ step 5

Smudge the eyeliner into the eyeshadow with a cotton swab so there are no hard lines and everything blends together. Drawing the eyeliner outward is easier; the line doesn't need to be solid as it will be smudged.

↑ step 6

Curl the eyelashes and apply mascara. For tips see page 102.

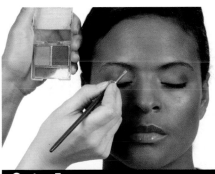

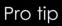 **↑ step 7**

To complete the eye look, groom and fill in the eyebrows (see page 112). Add blusher, natural-colored lipstick, and a touch of gloss.

Pro tip

Dark skin tones can also carry colorful eyeshadows well for evening and party looks.

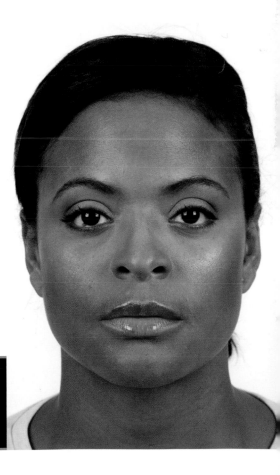

Blue eyes

➔ step 1

First apply foundation over the eyelid. Then brush nude matte shadow from the lash line to the brow as a blending base and to even the tone. Lighten under the arch of the brow with a paler eyeshadow. Apply soft gray shadow as a wash of color from the lash line to the crease.

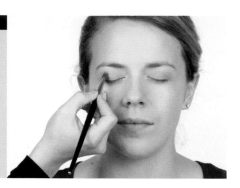

⬅ step 2

Softly line the eyes to give definition to the lashes. With a detail brush, apply a dark matte gray or black shadow along the top lash line and under the bottom lashes close to the roots of the lashes. Start at the outer corner and brush inward, making short strokes. It is harder to get a precise line in this direction, but powder is easier to apply than kohl (for eyeliner tips see page 99).

➔ step 3

Complete the eyes by curling the lashes and applying mascara. Groom and, if necessary, fill in the eyebrows (see page 112).

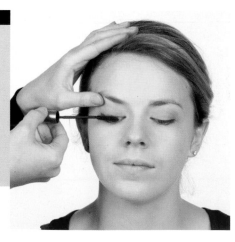

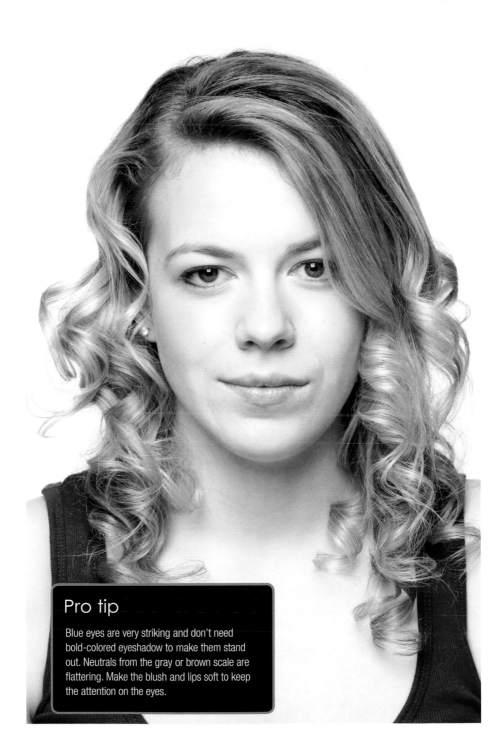

Pro tip

Blue eyes are very striking and don't need
bold-colored eyeshadow to make them stand
out. Neutrals from the gray or brown scale are
flattering. Make the blush and lips soft to keep
the attention on the eyes.

Green eyes

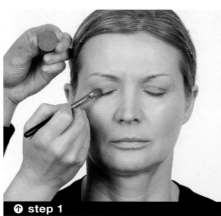

⬆ step 1

First apply foundation over the eyelid and then brush nude matte shadow from the lash line to the brow as a blending base and to even the tone. Lighten under the arch of the brow with a paler eyeshadow. Then apply a charcoal gray eyeshadow over the eyelids, from the lash line to the crease.

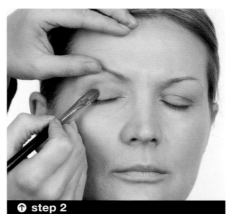

⬆ step 2

As we get older, the skin over the eyelid becomes looser and can crease as you brush over it so parts of the eyelid are missed. To ensure you cover the whole lid with shadow, lift the brow to pull the skin tighter and move the brush in small strokes inward and outward.

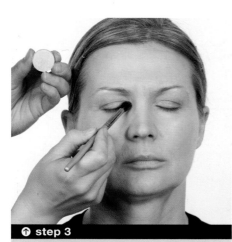

⬆ step 3

Apply a paler eyeshadow with a shimmer finish to the inner corner of the eyelid to highlight and open the eye.

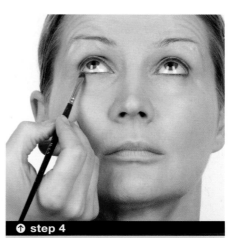

⬆ step 4

Define along the lower lash using a fine detail brush and charcoal powder. Apply under the lashes close to the roots, starting at the outer corner and making small strokes as you brush in toward the inner corner.

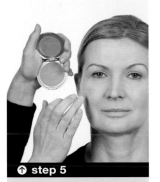

↑ step 5

For a natural look or a look on slightly older or drier skin, apply cream blush to the apples of the cheeks, blending with your fingers.

➔ step 6

Groom and fill the eyebrows to enhance the shape, or correct it if they are sparse, using brow powder or matte eyeshadow in a color that matches the natural hair color (see page 112). Curl the eyelashes and apply mascara.

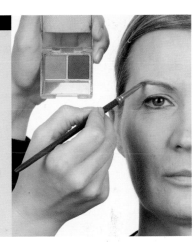

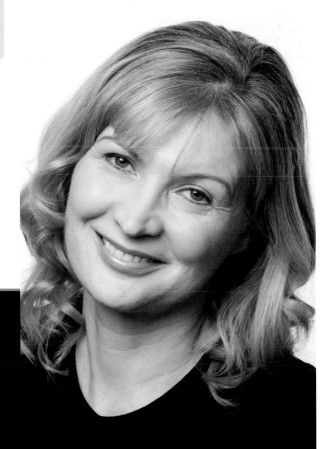

Pro tip

The green color in your eyes will really jump out if you use purple eyeshadow. Strong colors are not suitable for older women, but a hint of purple or mauve will have a similar effect.

Gray eyes

➔ step 1

Apply foundation over the eyelid as an eye base. Brush nude matte shadow all over the eyelids from the lash line to the brow, to help with blending and evening the tone of the eyelid. Lighten under the arch of the brow and inner corner with a paler eyeshadow to open the eye.

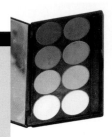

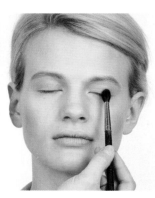

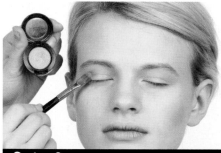

⬆ step 2

Brush pale green eyeshadow over the lid, and then enhance the color and the eyes by blending a slightly darker green over the outer third of the eyelid from the lash line up to and slightly above the crease. Blend inward, outward, and in small circles.

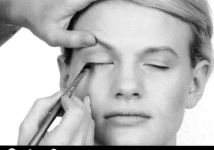

⬆ step 3

Line along the top lashes with brown kohl; the line should be very fine and close to the root of the lashes. Either use a pencil, with a sharp end for precision application, or a soft cream kohl or gel liner from a pot with a flat liner brush (see page 96). Draw the line from the outer corner inward, making small strokes.

➔ step 4

Apply a mid-brown matte shadow under the bottom lashes, at the roots. With a fine detail brush, start at the outer corner and work inward, making small strokes with the brush. Curl the lashes and apply mascara (see page 102). Add blush in a soft shade (see page 72) and lip gloss to complete the look.

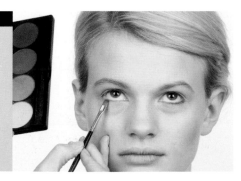

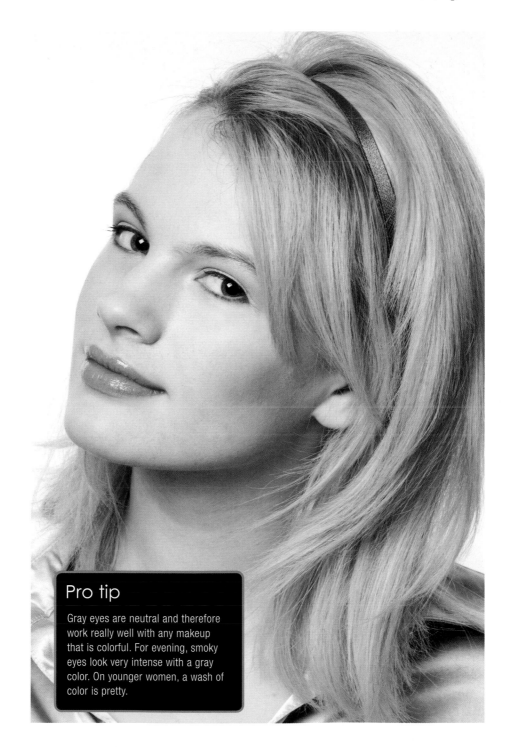

Pro tip

Gray eyes are neutral and therefore work really well with any makeup that is colorful. For evening, smoky eyes look very intense with a gray color. On younger women, a wash of color is pretty.

PARTY EYES

There will be times when the looks you feel comfortable creating just won't do for either the occasion or your mood. In this case a little extra something is needed, and adding glitter or using a bold color could be just that thing.

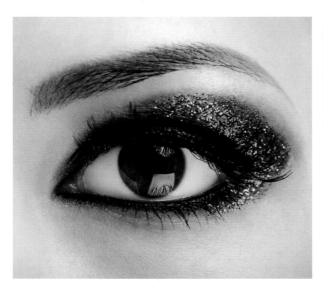

Pro tip

Eyes are the obvious feature to play up for a party look. A hint of glitter in silver, black, or gold along the lash line or outer third of the eyelid can be used to enhance a smoky eye, or you can go for a colored glitter and build the eye look around it. Experiment with bold colors, blending them over the eye; or for a different look, apply a solid block of intense color.

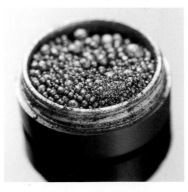

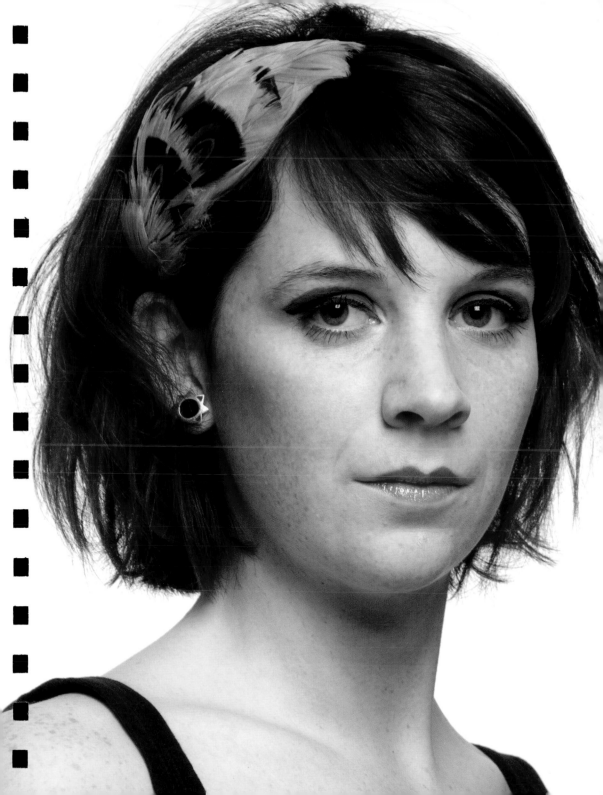

Using glitter

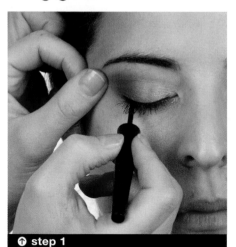

⬆ step 1

Follow steps 1 to 3 for a strong eye look (see page 138). Then line along the top lashes using liquid eyeliner. Pull your eyelid taut so the line is solid. The skin on your eyelid is loose and can ruffle up slightly, which can give a broken eye line.

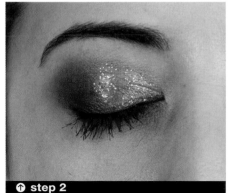

⬆ step 2

Apply glitter over the inner two-thirds of the eyelid. The easiest product to use and the one that will actually stay where you put it is glitter that is suspended in water or gel. It takes 15 seconds to dry so keep your eye closed until it is completely dry. Press the glitter onto the eyeshadow so that you don't disturb it.

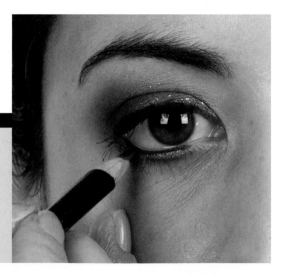

➔ step 3

Line inside the lower eyelid with a black kohl pencil. Pull the eyelid down slightly so it is away from the wetness of the eye and, making short strokes, line from the outer corner inward.

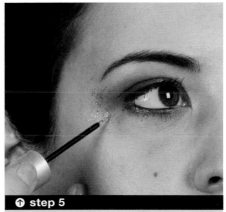

↑ step 4

To finish, curl the lashes and apply mascara to the top and bottom lashes.

↑ step 5

For additional sparkle, apply glitter as a highlight around the eye, on the cheekbone, and up toward the temple.

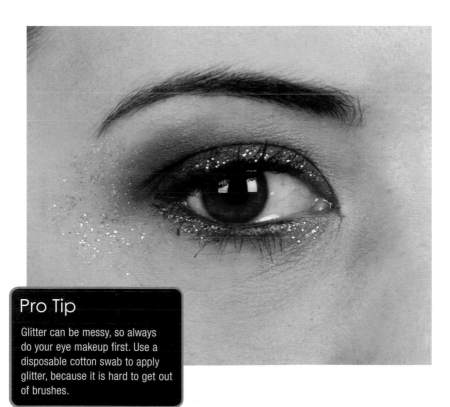

Pro Tip

Glitter can be messy, so always do your eye makeup first. Use a disposable cotton swab to apply glitter, because it is hard to get out of brushes.

LIPS

You have the basic skills to apply lipstick in a shade and shape that suit you. Now learn some variations for different occasions and outfits.

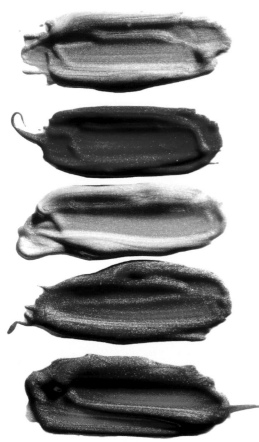

There are no rules as far as lips are concerned. Most women choose to keep colors lighter for daytime and darker for night. Matte and cream finishes offer a subtler look, while a high-gloss finish adds glamour. If in doubt, a sheer, natural-looking color with a little shine works well any time.

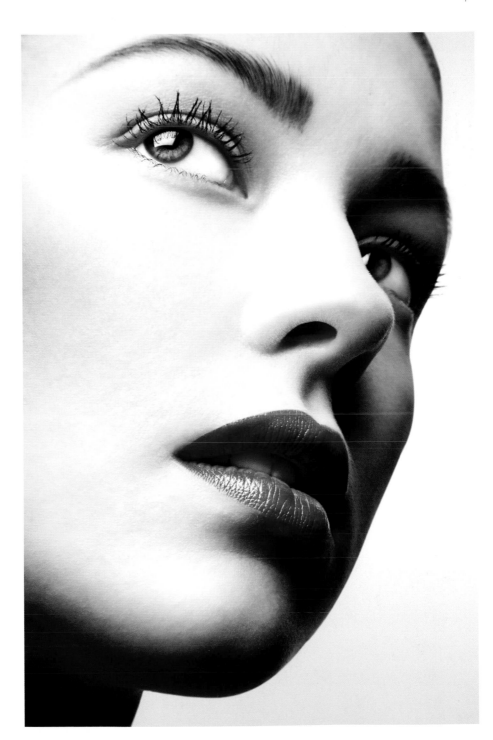

Light

For a long-lasting, defined lip, use lipliner first, then lipstick, even if you are using a natural color. Follow with gloss if you like shine. Filling the whole lip with the pencil will ensure an even application of color and increase the longevity of the color without the dry look of a matte lipstick.

➔ step 1

First outline the center of the top lips, across the bow of the lips, and then outline the center of the bottom lip.

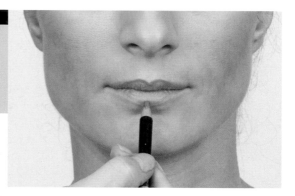

⬆ step 2

Lightly fill in the whole lip area with the pencil and then work the pencil into the lips with a lip brush.

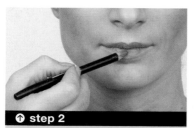

➔ step 3

Using a lip brush, apply nude lipstick. After applying it all over the lips, blot with a tissue and repeat the application.

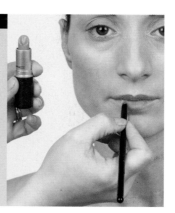

⬅ step 4

Add shine to the lips by applying clear lip gloss on top of the lipstick.

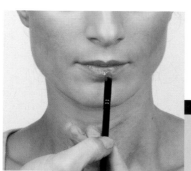

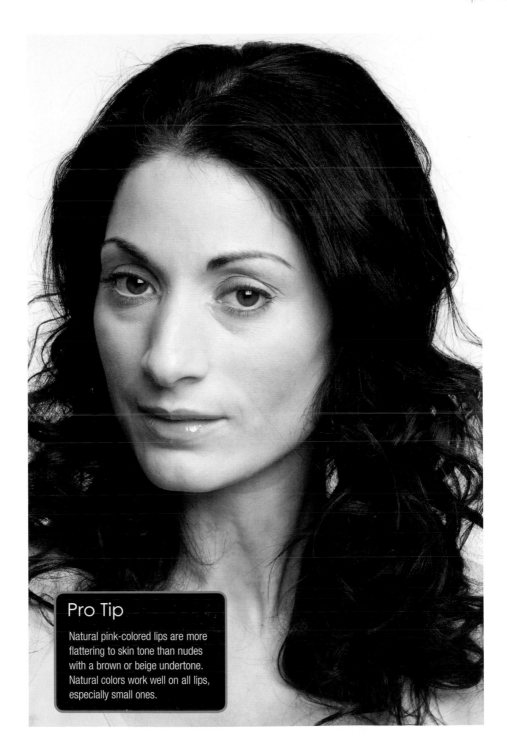

Pro Tip

Natural pink-colored lips are more flattering to skin tone than nudes with a brown or beige undertone. Natural colors work well on all lips, especially small ones.

Medium

Sometimes you need more than a natural lip to balance your makeup look.
If you are applying lipstick for an occasion when you will be photographed, a
medium color will come across well.

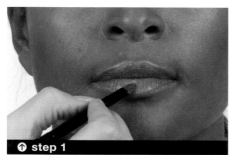

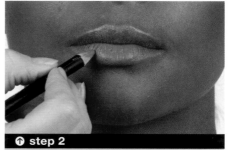

⬆ step 1

Before you start the rest of your makeup,
apply balm to the lips to soften them. It will
sink into the lips by the time you return to do
the lips and will give a good base for the lip
pencil to glide on smoothly.

⬆ step 2

To increase the staying power of the lipstick, fill
them with a pencil first. Start by applying pencil
to the outline in the center of the top and
bottom lips and then fill in (see page 168).
Sometimes the top and bottom lips vary in
color on dark skin tones. You can balance the
color by using a slightly lighter or darker pencil.

➔ step 3

Apply lipstick in a slightly
darker shade than the lipliner all
over the lips. Work the color
into the lips with a lip brush.
Blot the lips and apply a second
coat of lipstick. You can then
add gloss on top.

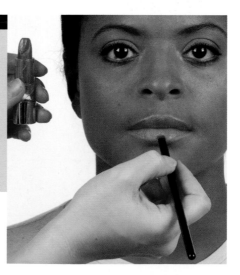

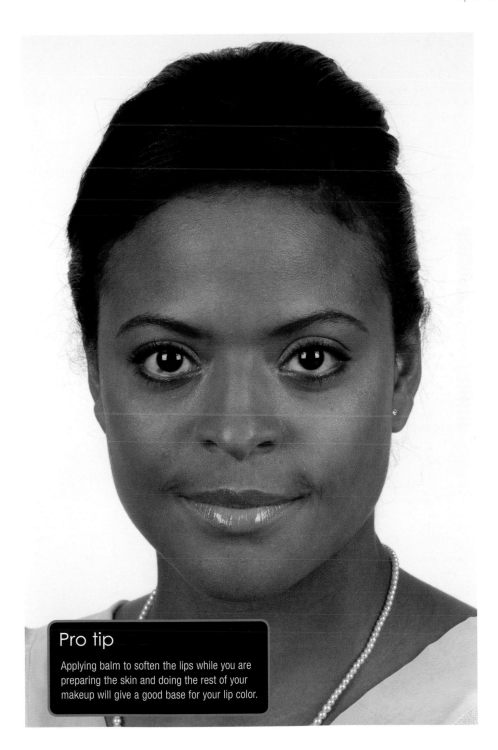

Pro tip

Applying balm to soften the lips while you are preparing the skin and doing the rest of your makeup will give a good base for your lip color.

Strong

It can be hard to get a perfect lip line with a dark pencil. If the line isn't clean or the lip shape is unbalanced, it can be hard to remove dark colors as they stain the lips. Use a neutral color to define the shape of the lips first and then apply a darker lip color on top.

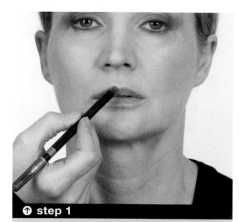

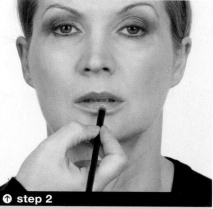

↑ step 1

It is a good idea to apply a product around the outside of the lip line that will stop the lipstick from bleeding. This is especially true on older skin. There are special products available or you can use concealer. Apply a shade that matches or is slightly lighter than your skin tone. Use a concealer brush around the outside of the lip line then line the lips with a neutral lipliner.

↑ step 2

Fill in the whole lip area with lip pencil; work it into the lips with a lip brush; and then blot with a tissue.

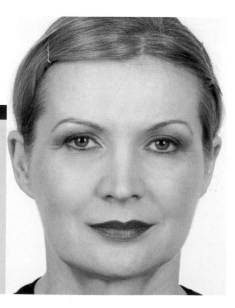

➔ step 3

Apply the strong color with a lip brush, building it up a little at a time until you are comfortable with the intensity. Take the color right up to the lip line, using a brush to give a more precise application. Blot the lipstick when you have gotten the required depth of color and then apply a thin layer on top for texture. Or, if you prefer a shiny finish, go for gloss. For even more intensity, choose a colored gloss.

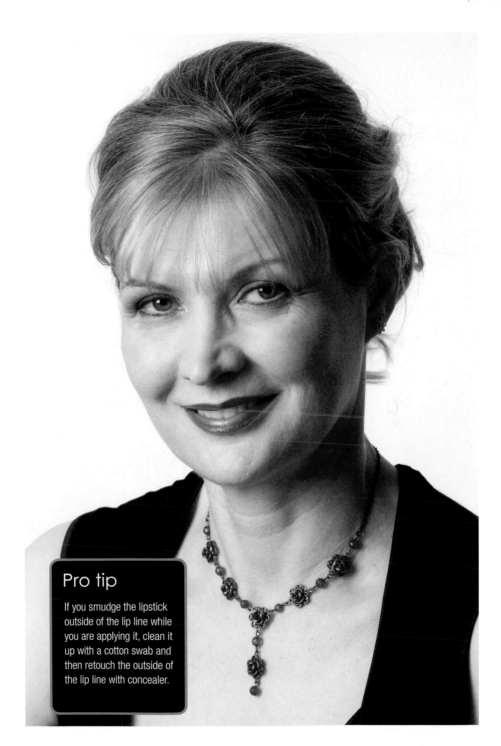

Pro tip

If you smudge the lipstick
outside of the lip line while
you are applying it, clean it
up with a cotton swab and
then retouch the outside of
the lip line with concealer.

Variations on lip looks

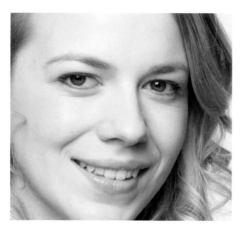

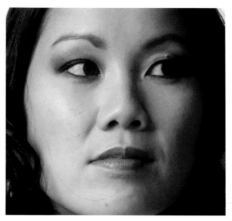

Blond hair and a fair complexion are brought to life with a fresh pink or coral-tinted balm or sheer lipstick. Use a slightly paler concealer around the outside of the lip line to enhance the shape.

For a professional look for a work event, important meeting, or even public speaking, choose a medium color that stands out but isn't too bold. Use a lip pencil over the lip first, and layer two coats of lipstick.

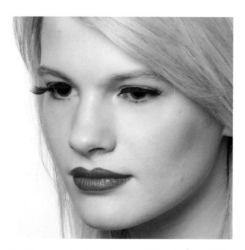

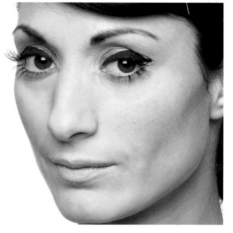

Red lips are classic and very striking. A matte finish is easier to wear, as it is less likely to bleed. The lip shape should be created with lip pencil. A steady hand is required to ensure symmetry.

Very pale, blanked-out lips have a period feel. They work well with strong eyes. Blush is required to add color to the complexion; otherwise, the lip color can be draining and will make you look ill.

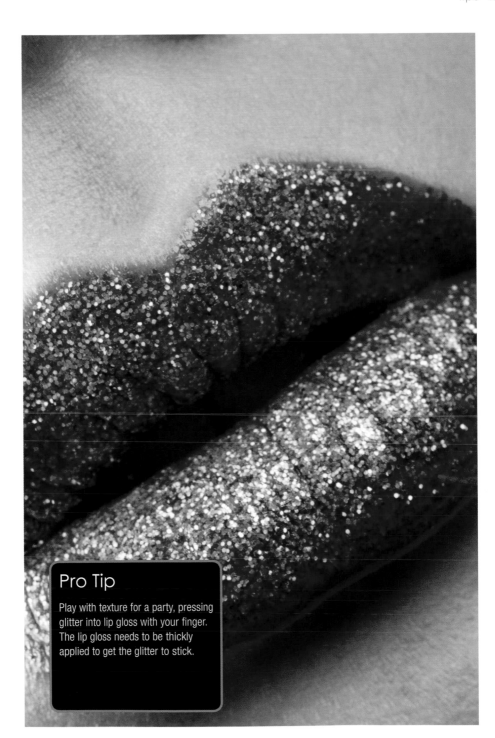

Pro Tip

Play with texture for a party, pressing glitter into lip gloss with your finger. The lip gloss needs to be thickly applied to get the glitter to stick.

CHEEKS

You can change your shade of blush to suit the season, changes in your skin tone, or an outfit. It is really important to learn the basics, and then you can combine contouring and highlighting with blush application. As with all makeup, a professional finish is obtained by building up the depth of color slowly and blending.

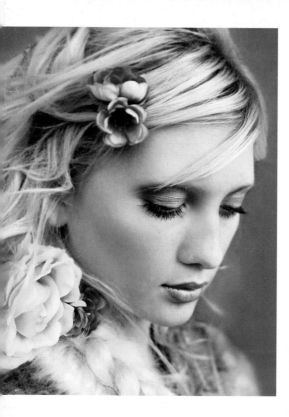

Color on your cheeks brings a freshness and glow to your complexion, making you look healthy and radiant. Color can be applied in different places to enhance or play up your features and face shapes. If you insist on having only two blushes in your makeup bag, don't choose two that are too similar. Go for a contrasting color and texture so you don't get stuck in a rut and then you can vary the shade between daytime and evening, summer and winter.

Pro tip

The tool you use to apply blush can dramatically change the end result. Invest in a good-quality brush to apply powder blush and keep it clean. A brush full of old product will give a patchy application.

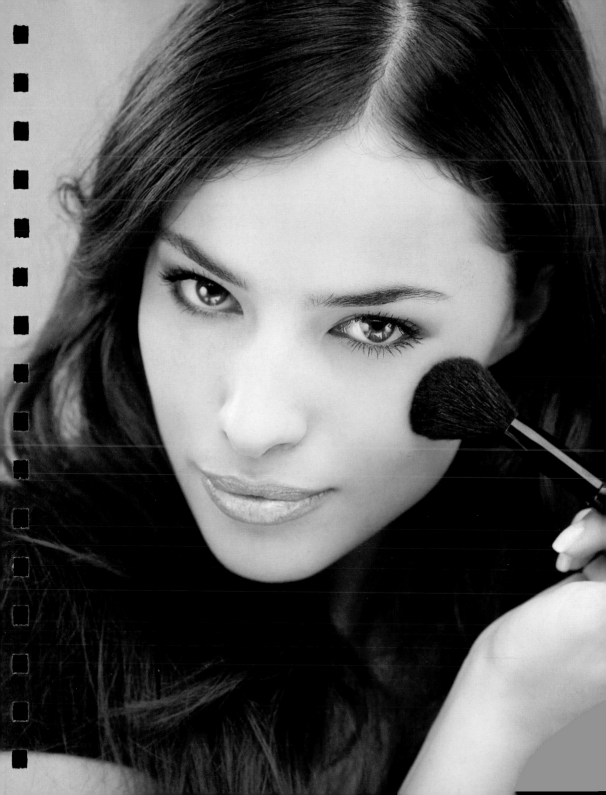

Products

There are many shades of blush available, from very natural to rich strong color, with various finishes such as matte or shimmer. The most common formulas are powder, liquid, and cream. The placement of the blush is explained on pages 72–4. For extra impact and a long-lasting finish, layer blush starting with cream and applying a powder in a similar shade on top.

Powder blush

Powder blush is easy to apply and comes in a huge range of colors. A more expensive product with stronger pigment will give a better finish. As well as using it on the cheeks, dusting powder blush on the temples enhances a healthy glow.

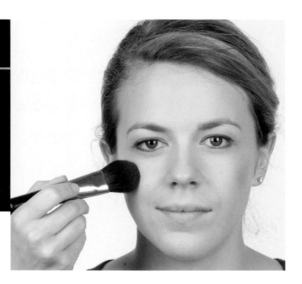

Cream blusher

Highly portable and great for the summer, cream blush is very versatile. It can be used on lips and eyes, as well as cheeks. No tools are required for applying, just fingers. Look for formulas that are creamy and not too dry.

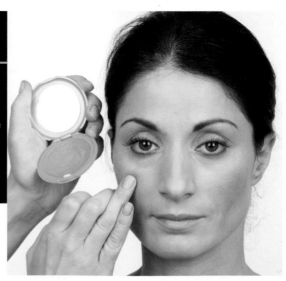

Warm beige Good for contouring medium skin tones and can be used as a bronzer. Doesn't have a deep enough color to impact on darker tones.

Warm apricot Gives a natural glow to Mediterranean skin tones, and is great in summer on slightly tanned skin.

Pale beige Perfect for shading fair and pale skin, for a subtle result. The color is too light for other skin tones.

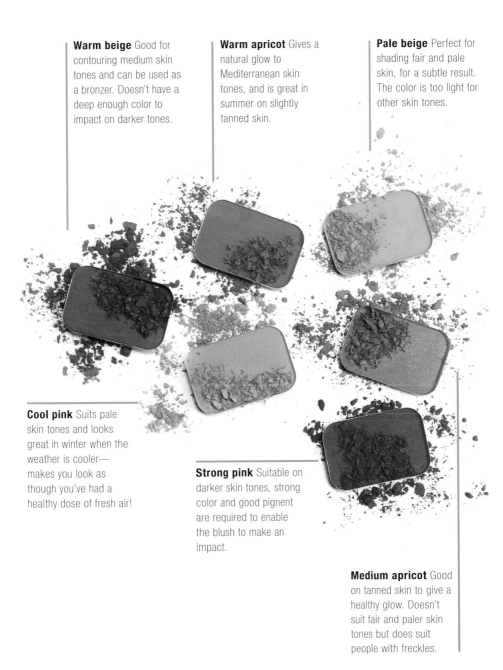

Cool pink Suits pale skin tones and looks great in winter when the weather is cooler— makes you look as though you've had a healthy dose of fresh air!

Strong pink Suitable on darker skin tones, strong color and good pigment are required to enable the blush to make an impact.

Medium apricot Good on tanned skin to give a healthy glow. Doesn't suit fair and paler skin tones but does suit people with freckles.

Making more impact

Step outside of your comfort zone and try bolder blush application to make cheeks a feature.

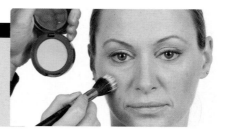

➔ step 1

Rather than going straight to a strong color first, swirl a more natural color over the apples of your cheeks and along your cheekbones.

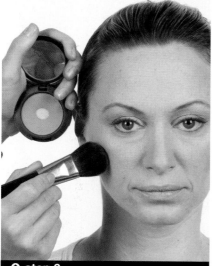

↑ step 2

Next add a stronger, bolder color from the same family, to give impact on the high points on the apples and top of the cheekbones.

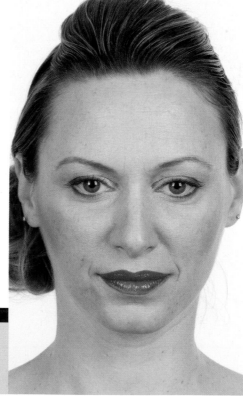

➔ step 3

Applied with a light touch and blended well, the end result is very striking and will have staying power. Apply lipstick in a striking red to balance the cheeks.

Using cream and powder

On darker skin tones where stronger color is required to make the blush stand out, or for real impact on lighter skin tones, layer cream and powder blush.

➔ step 1

First apply cream blush with your fingers or a small fiber-optic brush.

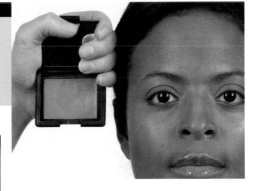

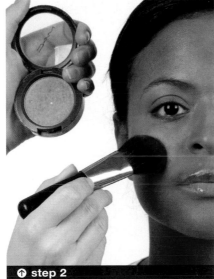

⬆ step 2

Brush a powder blush on top. Use a color with the same depth and intensity as the cream blush on dark skin tones; use a lighter-colored powder on fairer skin tones.

➔ step 3

Layering a powder on top of a cream blush will really make the color stand out—just make sure you blend well.

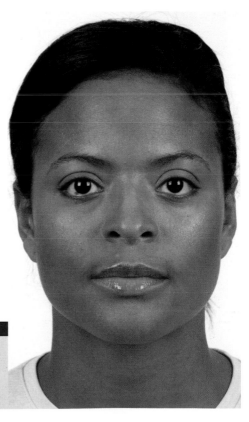

BRIDAL MAKEUP

There are many things to consider when planning your wedding, and your makeup is no exception. You will be wearing probably the most glamourous and expensive dress you will ever own and you will be the center of attention. Your makeup needs to reflect all of this. It also needs to not be overwhelming when you are talking to someone face-to-face, but it should still make an impact when someone is looking at you from across the room. Bridal makeup and evening makeup are not the same thing; bridal makeup needs to be durable, should be classic; and ought to be suitable for photographs.

When I ask a bride what she wants to look like on her wedding day, most say they want to look like themselves but better. They don't want to startle the groom by being much more made-up than they normally are, but they want the makeup to stand out in photographs.

Striking this balance can be tricky, especially if you are doing your makeup yourself. I always start a bridal consultation by asking questions about the day and the bride's normal makeup routine. By thinking about these things yourself, you will achieve a makeup look that works.

To stand out in photographs, makeup doesn't need to be heavy or dramatic, but it needs to be well applied with features that are well-defined. It is important that the texture of the skin is smooth but not shiny.

Before the big day

It is important you look after your skin in the months prior to your wedding to help you look radiant on the big day. I recommend evaluating your skincare routine and making the necessary changes six months before. If you don't have that much time, it's never too late to make a difference. Book yourself a facial, then ask for and take advice from your beauty therapist. He or she will be able to recommend products and a beauty regime. Now is the time to invest in a good cleanser and moisturizer. Don't do anything radical or different too close to the wedding.

Exercise, diet, and drinking water will affect the quality of your skin. Cut down on coffee and alcohol, replacing them with fruit smoothies, water, or herbal tea. Exfoliate regularly; this removes dead skin cells and leaves your skin feeling smooth and vibrant.

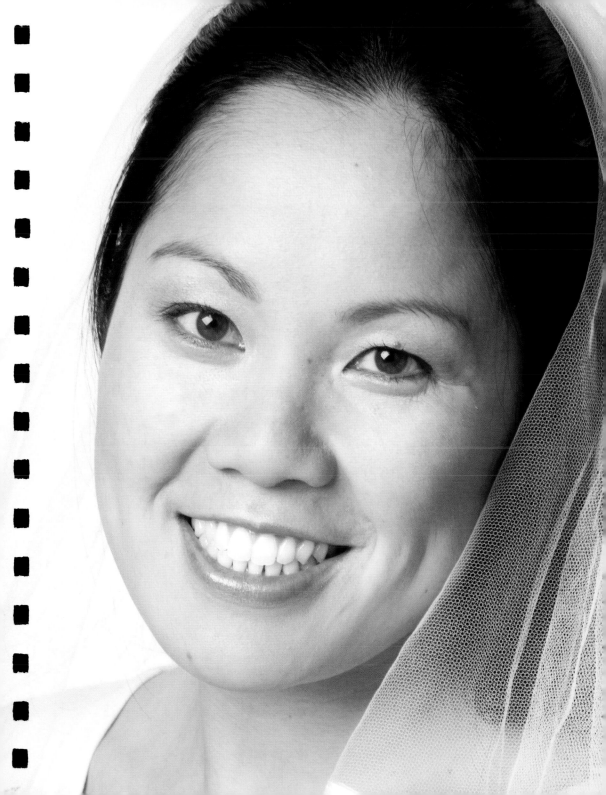

PRACTICAL CONSIDERATIONS

Whether you are having your makeup done professionally or doing it yourself, you should consider:

- Time of day—midday sunshine, evening?
- Season—winter, summer, inside or out?
- Weather—bright sunshine, overcast?
- Style and color of your dress and your bridesmaids' dresses—everything should work in harmony together. For instance, if your bridesmaids wear silver and you have a small amount of silver in your eyeshadow, it will be enhanced when you stand next to them.
- Hairstyle—are you going formal or loose?

Don't go for high fashion or bright colors. Makeup should be classic and understated. Timeless is hard to achieve, as what we think is a timeless look today won't be timeless in 20 years; fashion moves on and tastes evolve. Keep in mind that both your face shape and skin type are important considerations for your makeup.

Eyes—Soft grays and browns are classic and suit everyone.
Cheeks—Define them, not too much bronzer.
Eyebrows—Frame the face.
Lips—Soft pink lipstick looks nice in photographs.
Face—Foundation should be the right color for luminous skin.

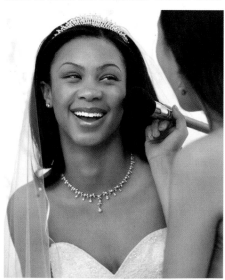

I start a bridal consultation by asking about someone's normal makeup routine, what they wear during the day, what they wear for a night out at a party. I ask people to bring reference pictures of makeup they like; bridal magazines and the red carpet pictures found in most women's magazines or on the Internet are excellent reference tools.

On the day allow plenty of time and make sure you have a well lit location set aside for doing your makeup, preferably in daylight. If you are doing your makeup yourself, make sure you have the right tools. Get a makeover at a professional department store makeup counter first, and tell the makeup artist it is for your wedding as they will be able to advise you; treat yourself to new products and practice using these a couple of times before the big day.

Choosing a professional makeup artist

A professional makeup artist is trained in techniques for face structure and color theory, and will have a professional kit of tried and tested products. Look for someone who is used to applying makeup for photography. Ask to see examples of their work from previous weddings and their professional portfolio, and ask for references from previous brides. Go on recommendations from friends or on bridal shows.

Have a trial run beforehand and don't be afraid to give feedback on the makeup. It is as much for the makeup artist as it is for you. One person's idea of a smoky eye is not the same as someone else's. The purpose of the trial is to make sure you are both singing from the same song sheet!

Other people

Bridesmaids should not outshine you, but the colors you choose should work with the color of their outfits and the colors in the bouquets.

It can be very hard to tell your friends to change their makeup if you don't like their normal style. If you are quite a natural makeup wearer and so are the majority of your bridesmaids, one who applies it with a trowel will really throw the balance and stand out in group photographs. A makeup artist is often the best person to try to steer them in the right direction and can help you both come to a compromise.

I often come across older women who do not wear makeup. If you are the mother of the bride and wish to make an extra effort on the day of the wedding, you can take years off and give yourself a new lease of life by evening out your skin tone, bringing color to your cheeks, and defining your eyes. Don't go overboard; for photographs a little makeup will make a big difference.

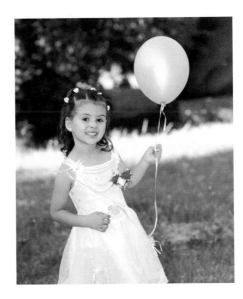

Dos and don'ts

- Refrain from having a cosmetic facial or facial hair removal at least two weeks before the wedding to avoid any irritation, allergies, puffiness, or redness. Also keep in mind that waxing temporarily changes the skin's texture and causes it to appear shiny, making your makeup more difficult to unify.
- The brows frame the eyes and it's important not to overpluck them. Take advice from your makeup artist and see a professional to re-shape them. If stray hairs appear on your big day, plucking one or two shouldn't be a problem.
- Drink lots of water in the final days before the wedding to give your face a healthy and vibrant appearance. Drinking water also flushes out toxins and can reduce bloating.
- Try to relax as much as possible the night before the wedding. You will want to be rested and ready on your wedding day. Have a warm bath with your favorite bath products nearby, light some fragrant candles, have some sleepy tea or a glass of wine, and enjoy your last night as a single girl!

Light bridal makeup

Vary this look with stronger colors depending on what you want to achieve, and replace any of the steps with other sections from this book if you want, but make sure you try any variations out on your own at home well in advance of your big day.

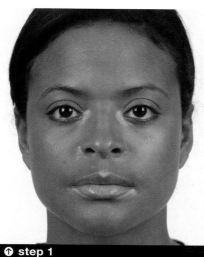

↑ step 1

On your wedding day you really need your makeup to last, so it is essential you prepare your skin properly before you start applying your makeup.

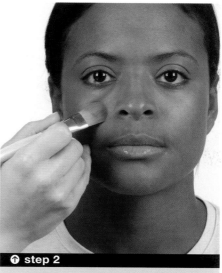

↑ step 2

Apply foundation, making sure you are using the correct shade. Start in the center and blend outward. Use a brush for an even application.

➜ step 3

Conceal around the eyes and cover any blemishes or redness. Use a concealer brush and tap into place with the pad of your middle finger (see page 52).

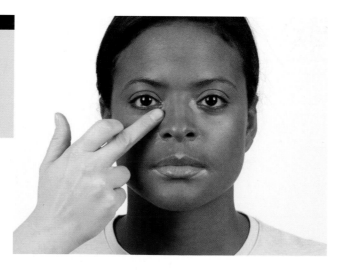

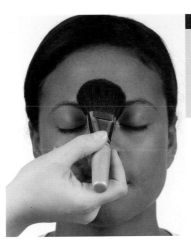

step 4

Apply powder to set the foundation and concealer. This is really important as you don't want to look shiny in pictures, and the powder will help the longevity of the makeup. Pile some loose powder onto the cheekbones to catch any falling eyeshadow.

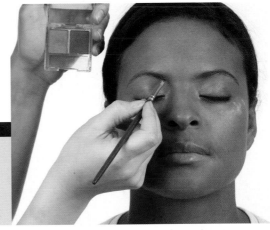

step 5

To frame the eyes and balance the whole face, groom and fill the eyebrows if necessary with brow gel or clear mascara to set them in place.

step 6

Start the eyes with an eye base for a long-lasting look and to neutralize the color of the eyelids from lash line to brows. Although it seems like a lot of layers and products, using a cream base will really help keep the eyeshadow crease-free.

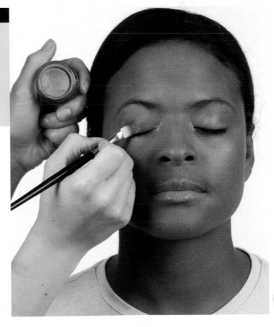

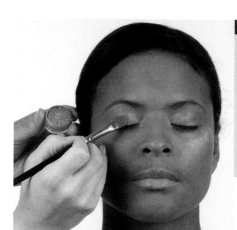

← step 7

step 7

Dust with a nude matte eyeshadow to set, using a similar color to the skin tone. Apply a complementary shimmer over the eyelid from the lashes to the crease. If it is loose, press it into the eyelid.

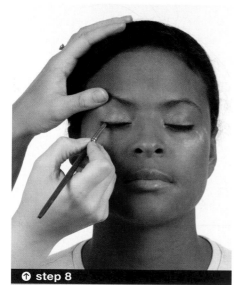

↑ step 8

Apply black liner along the lash line to enhance the lash and give definition to the eyes. This will make them stand out in photographs and give impact from a distance.

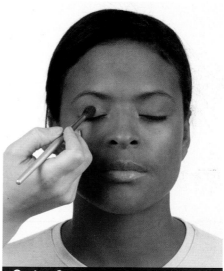

↑ step 9

Apply a darker brown color onto the outer third of the eyelid, blending into and slightly above the crease. Blend well with a blending brush.

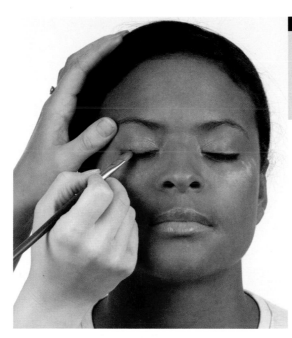

⬅ step 10

Smudge the dark brown eyeshadow into the lash line to soften the liner.

⬅ step 11

Blend lightly with a cotton swab.

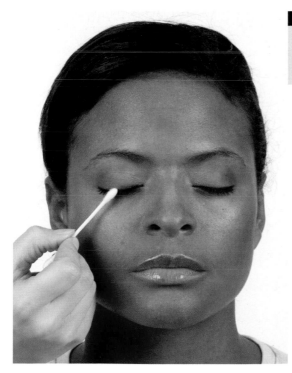

Pro tips

- Remember: If you want to make this look stronger, balance the different elements. Strong lips require a bit more blush applied to the apples of the cheeks.
- Add a dab of white shimmer in the cupid's bow to enhance the shape of the lips.

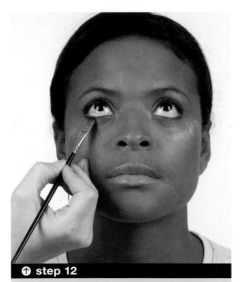

↑ step 12

With a detail brush, apply dark brown eyeshadow along the bottom lash line, close to the root of the lashes. Curl the eyelashes and apply mascara.

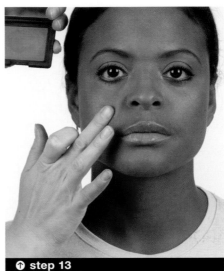

↑ step 13

For a long-wearing blush application and to make the color "pop," first apply cream blush with your finger to the apples of the cheeks.

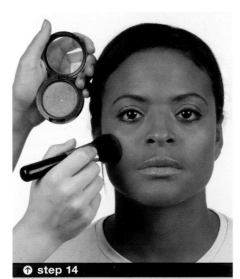

↑ step 14

With a blush brush, apply powder blush in the same color on top of the cream blusher. See page 68 for blush placement tips.

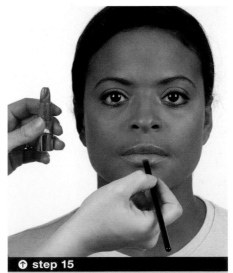

↑ step 15

On your wedding day you want really well-applied, long-lasting lip color. Remember you will kiss a lot of people! Start with lipliner all over the lips and then apply lipstick in a similar shade.

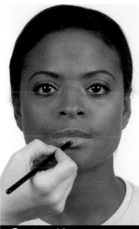

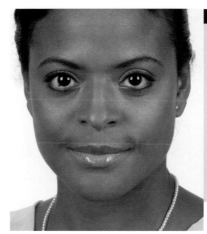

⬆ step 16

Really work the lipstick into the lips with a lip brush, and blot the lipstick two or three times. Reapply.

⬅ step 17

To give the lips texture, add a touch of gloss in the center. Don't apply too much, as it will smudge the lipstick and is not long-wearing. Take the gloss with you for touch-ups.

Pro tip

If you want to make this look stronger, balance the different elements. Strong lips require a touch more blush applied to the apples of the cheeks.

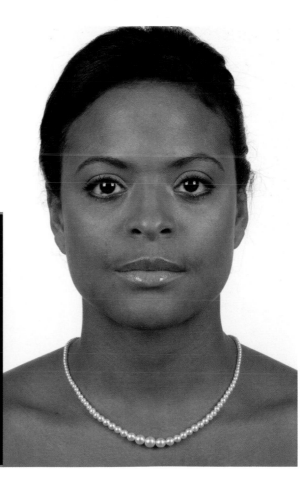

Variations on a bridal look

There are no rules for your wedding day. I would advise taking the makeup up one notch from what you usually wear, keeping a classic image in mind.

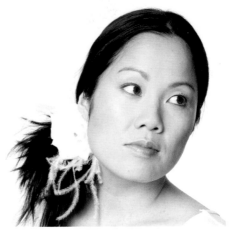

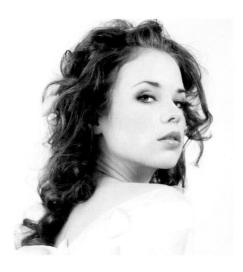

A natural look is timeless. Focus on clear, clean skin with softly defined features, and everyone will comment on how radiant you look.

Smoky eyes can be striking. I would advise getting a professional to do them for you and don't go overboard.

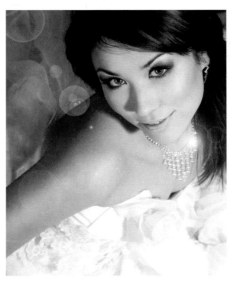

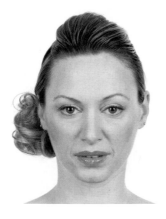

A strong look works well for a wedding that is later in the day or for a winter wedding when most of your photographs will be taken inside.

There is a middle ground between natural and smoky. Enhance the cheeks and lips, while keeping the eyes defined but not too heavy.

➲ Instead of using browns and grays, colors in the pink and auburn range can really complement the whites, ivories, and champagnes of wedding dresses.

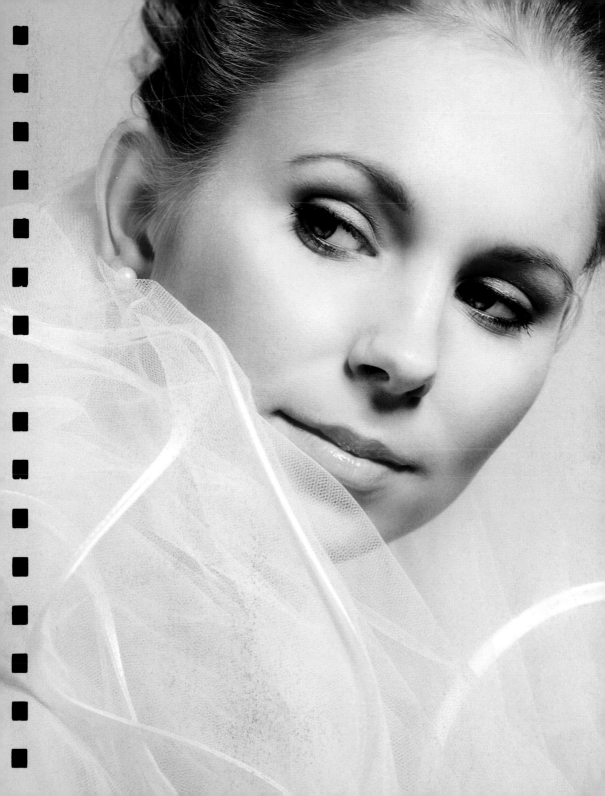

Chapter 4

APPLYING MAKEUP TO OTHERS

Whether your best friend needs a hand getting ready
for a big date, or your kids and their friends need
entertaining during school vacation, here are useful
ideas and practical considerations for you.

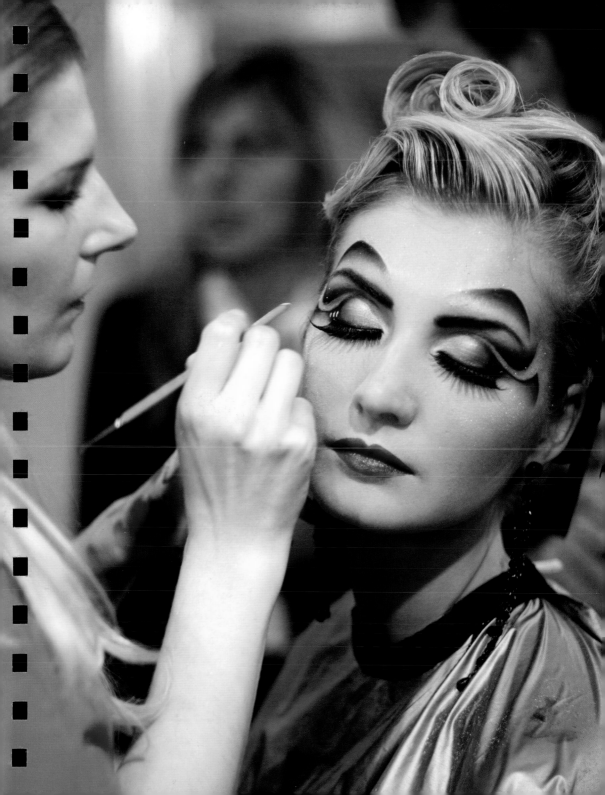

PRACTICAL CONSIDERATIONS

If you are going to apply makeup to someone else, you need to consider the following:

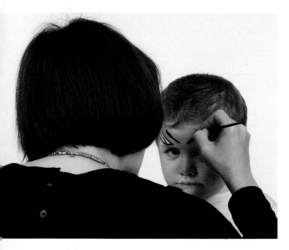

- The right tools for the job. You should have a good set of professional brushes and they need to be clean. You may also need puffs, sponges, tissues, cotton swabs, and makeup wipes.
- As soon as you start to apply makeup to someone else, hygiene and safety become your responsibility. You should ensure there is no chance of passing on infection or cross-contamination from unclean tools or products such as mascara.
- Where you are going to apply the makeup. You should have a chair to sit the person in that is a good height and won't hurt your back. They should sit in front of a mirror, and you should have good light, preferably daylight.
- Do you have a wide enough range of colors to suit every skin tone? To be safe, ask the person to bring his or her own foundation and concealer.
- If you are applying the makeup for a special occasion such as a wedding, make sure you have a practice session beforehand.

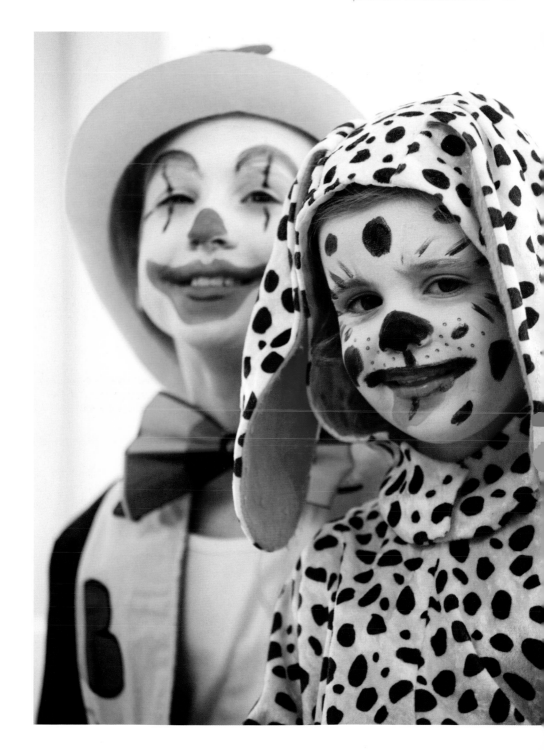

MEN

A good skincare routine is just as important for you as it is for women. Help yourself look your best by following the advice below.

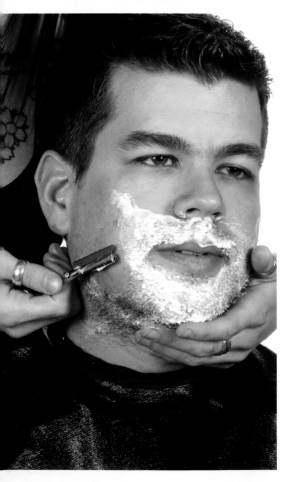

Most men look after their skin for exactly the same reason women do—to slow down the visible effects of aging and to increase the healthy appearance of their skin. It is not uncommon anymore for men to have a skincare routine, and more and more products are being developed for men.

There are a lot of men who have not picked up on this trend yet, so you can be a huge help to your friends or partner by educating them! Men shouldn't look after their skin only to counteract aging. The skin is the body's shield that protects it from germs and diseases.

There are a variety of situations in which you might wear makeup. A small but growing number of men use it daily to enhance their complexion and cover blemishes, dark circles, or imperfections on the surface of the skin. If you are appearing on television, in a film, on the stage, or in a photoshoot, makeup is required; the strongest makeup requirement is for the stage where features need to be visible from a distance. For other situations makeup should be very subtle and you should not look like you are wearing any. The makeup steps shown for applying makeup on the next few pages would be suitable for a theatrical performance—for other situations these steps can be followed but they should be toned down considerably.

The difference between men and women

- Men's skin starts to age slightly later than women's, as it contains more elastin and collagen.
- Men's skin is thicker and firmer.
- Men's pores are larger.
- Men's skin is drier, mainly due to shaving every day.

From these points you can see right away what to do for your skin. You will need a heavier moisturizer to counteract the dryness and to penetrate through the thicker layers. It is also important for you to clean your skin to control the surface oiliness and stop pores from getting blocked.

When men's skin ages, the combination of the skin thinning and the higher levels of collagen reducing at the same time means it is prone to getting deeper wrinkles than women's skin is. It is a good idea for men to use an eye cream, applied in the same way as for women.

Men should always cleanse to purify their skin before shaving, and moisturize after shaving. It is also important you use protection against sun damage during the day if you are outside a lot.

Male eyebrow grooming

If your eyebrows are a good length and sit neatly over each eye with a space over your nose, you've probably not paid much attention to them. However if someone has bushy eyebrows, a monobrow, or worse, has had them shaved off, it will be the first thing that catches someone's eye.

Grooming your brows, banishing a monobrow, or trimming the stray long ends, will make a huge difference to your overall appearance. To groom them at home, try trimming or tweezing. You will need a mirror, preferably a magnifying one, small sharp scissors, and a good pair of tweezers.

- Most of the time all that will be required is to trim a few stray hairs. Trim the hairs in the direction of hair growth. Be careful not to cut the hairs too short as they will stick out.
- The next step is plucking your eyebrows. This can be painful if your tweezers aren't sharp. The ideal time to pluck stray hairs is after a shower, as the warm water and steam will open the pores and make it easier. Tweeze in the direction of hair growth and pull one hair at a time.

If you have a monobrow and aren't sure where each brow should start, follow the steps on page 112. When you are grooming your brows, don't remove or trim too many hairs. Work with the natural shape of the brows. If you are not confident about shaping or trimming, go to a professional. Never shave your eyebrows; you will regret it afterward.

Makeup for men

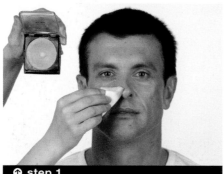

⬆ step 1

Using a sponge, apply a light cream-based foundation in a tone that matchs the skincolor. Working from the bridge of the nose, blend outward in all directions toward the perimeter of the face.

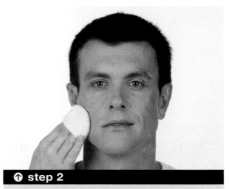

⬆ step 2

Press translucent loose powder into the skin to control shine and set the foundation, then dust over the top with a clean powder brush to remove any excess.

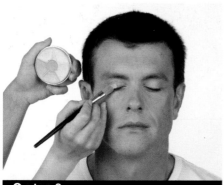

⬆ step 3

Use concealer to cover any darkness around the eyes, blemishes, or redness. To enhance the shape of the eyes and make them appear bigger, lightly blend a lighter shade of concealer or foundation over the eyelid from the lashes to the crease.

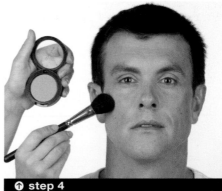

⬆ step 4

To give definition to the face, lightly shade under the cheekbones with a matte powder one shade darker than the skin tone. Never use a product that contains shimmer.

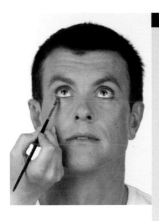

⬅ step 5

To enhance the shape of the eyes, shade along the top and bottom lash lines very close to the root of the lashes with a brown matte eyeshadow. If the eyebrows are thin or uneven, fill them with the same shadow, using a slanted eyeshadow brush. This should all be done very subtly.

Pro Tips

- You can use shading to reduce a receding hair line or large forehead by using matte contouring blush, one or two shades darker than the skin tone.
- You can use shading to minimize a double chin by using matte contouring blush two shades darker than the skin tone. Apply subtly and blend well.
- Cover any redness on the neck caused by shaving. First try covering with foundation; but if the coverage is not heavy enough, use concealer. Blend the edges well and match to the tone of the surrounding skin.
- Moisten dry lips with lip balm, but don't use anything glossy or shiny.
- It is possible to cover the beard line with heavier foundation if required, but don't apply heavy foundation all over the face as it will look like a mask. Just increase the coverage in the required area.
- A wide nose can be slimmed with shading (see page 66).
- If the skin is pale or you look particularly tired, the complexion can be warmed up with the addition of a matte bronzer.

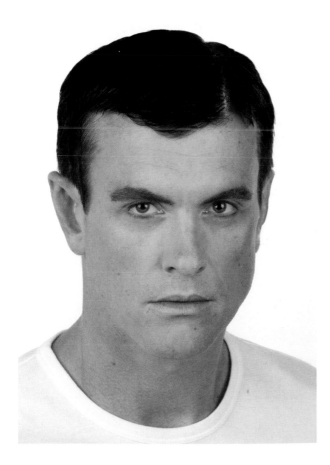

CHILDREN

Washable face paints are a must for children—suitable for a party or just to kill some time during school vacation. Your children will love these designs, which are endlessly customizable.

Face painting

➔ step 1

Paint the face white using white face paint applied with a sponge.

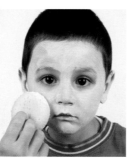

➔ step 2

Paint the eye sockets black.

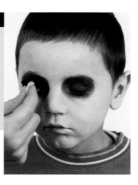

↑ step 3

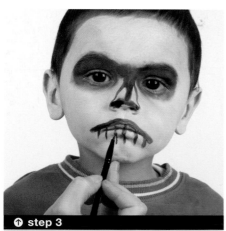

Using a thin synthetic brush, paint black on the nose and draw a scary mouth.

↑ step 4

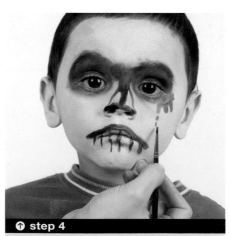

To finish, add red face paint dripping from one eye socket.

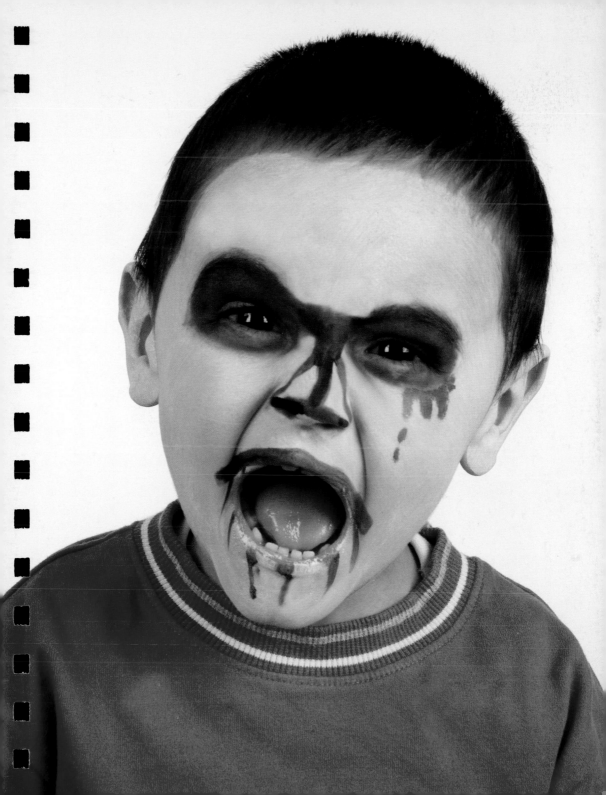

Face painting

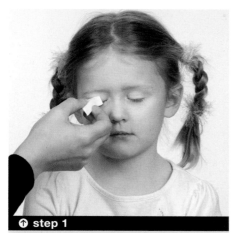

↑ step 1

Using plain white face paint, cover the eye area.

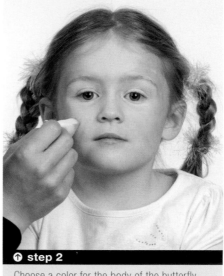

↑ step 2

Choose a color for the body of the butterfly and apply it, using the rounded side of a sponge in a sweeping motion around each eye to give wing shapes.

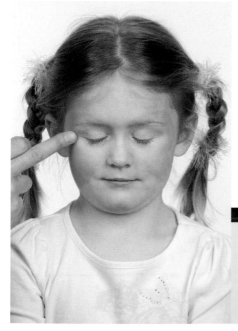

← step 3

To highlight the center of the wings, paint a contrasting lighter color over the eye area. I have used yellow, blending it out into the pink to give three different colors. Any bright colors can be used to create this face paint.

→ step 4

With a small synthetic brush, outline the wing shapes in purple, using short strokes to create a scalloped edge.

For the body of the butterfly, paint dots down the center of the nose with a synthetic brush. Start at the top and make the dots smaller as you move down the nose.

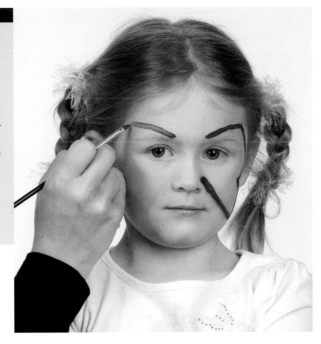

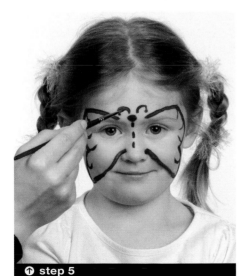

↑ step 5

From the top dot, add two curly antennae to finish the head.

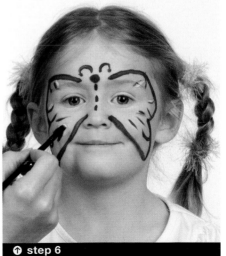

↑ step 6

Decorate the wings by painting on swirls and adding glitter.

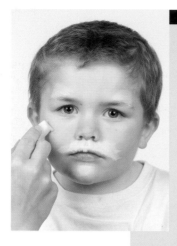

⬅ step 1

Paint white face paint around the mouth using a sponge. With a clean sponge, paint yellow face paint around the eyes, cheeks, and chin. Paint two white triangles above the eyes. Use the line of the actual eyebrow as a guide.

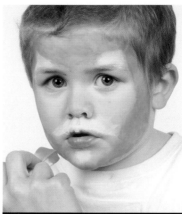

⬆ step 2

Rinse the sponge and add orange around the outside of the face. Blend the orange and yellow together by going slightly over the edges of the yellow paint with the orange.

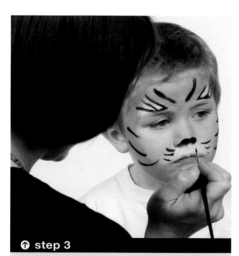

⬆ step 3

Starting your brush strokes at the outer edge of the orange paint and dragging inward, add black whiskers and stripes and highlight with white around the mouth and on the sides of the face.

Using the black face paint, add a nose, painting onto the tip of the actual nose.

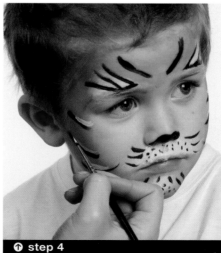

⬆ step 4

Using a thin brush, add small black dots above the top lip and outline the whiskers and eyebrows to give more definition.

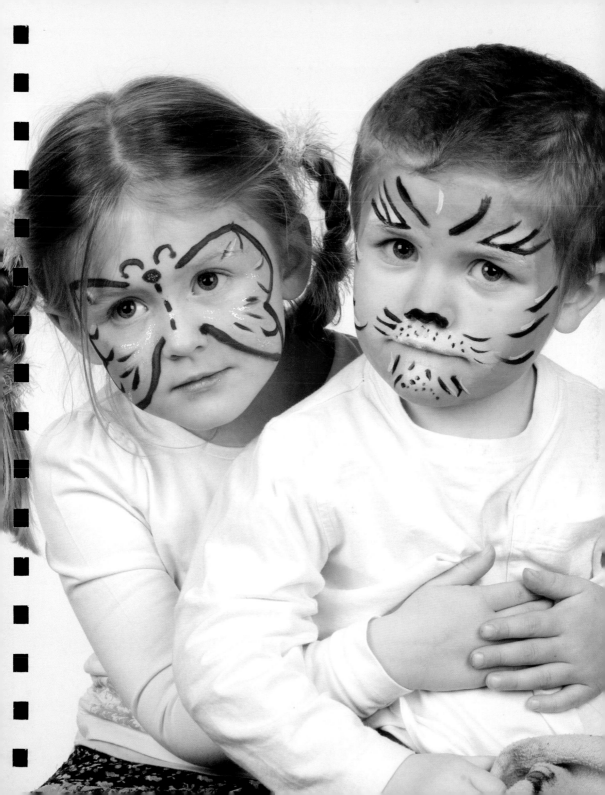

COSTUME PARTY

The following techniques can be modified to suit other themes and occasions, but will give you an idea of how to achieve a range of makeup-based effects.

Costume party gore

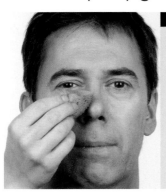

◐ step 1

Apply a green water-based face paint all over the face, starting around the edges. Dip your sponge in water as you do the center of the face so it is paler.

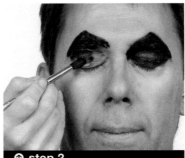

↑ step 2

Cover the eyelids with black face paint.

➔ step 3

Paint black face paint through the eyebrows and above in a triangle shape to overemphasize the eyebrows.

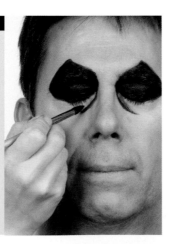

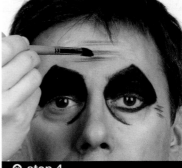

↑ step 4

Dirty the forehead by smudging black paint in with your finger.

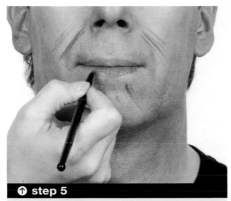

↑ step 5

Using a detail brush, paint lines in creases under the eyes and in other places where you see fit.

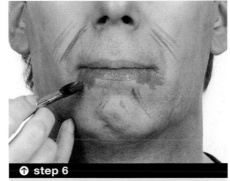

↑ step 6

Paint lips red and add dripping blood to the corners.

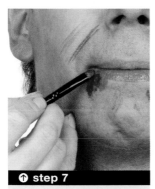

↑ step 7

Go over with fake blood for a more gruesome effect.

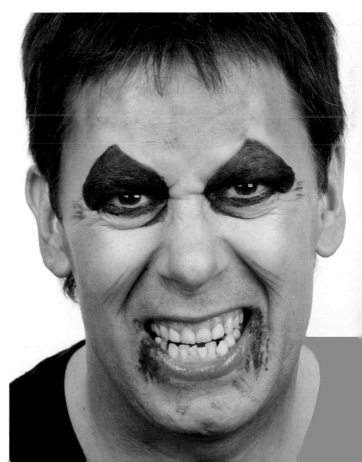

Costume party fantasy

➔ step 1

Use a strong green all over each eyelid from the lashes to the eyebrows. For a deeper color, use greasepaint (theatrical makeup) rather than face paint.

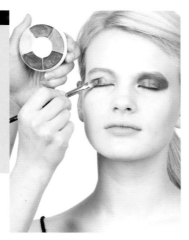

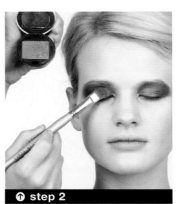

⬆ step 2

Set grease by pressing powder shadow into it. Apply green along the bottom lash line.

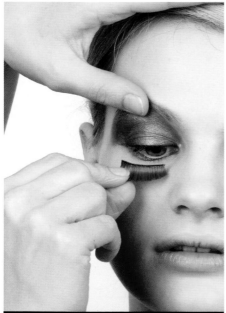

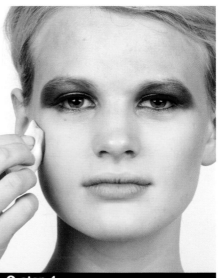

⬆ step 3

Apply fake lashes (see page 95).

⬆ step 4

Using a sponge, blend green over the forehead and the sides of the face.

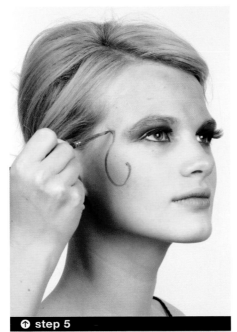

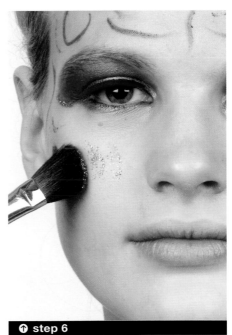

↑ step 5

Paint swirls on the cheeks.

↑ step 6

Highlight the swirls with glitter.

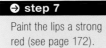

⊙ step 7

Paint the lips a strong
red (see page 172).

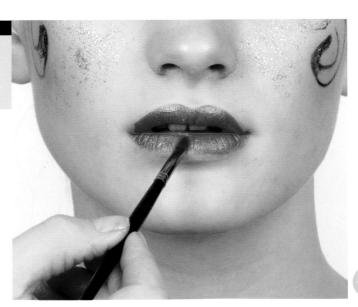

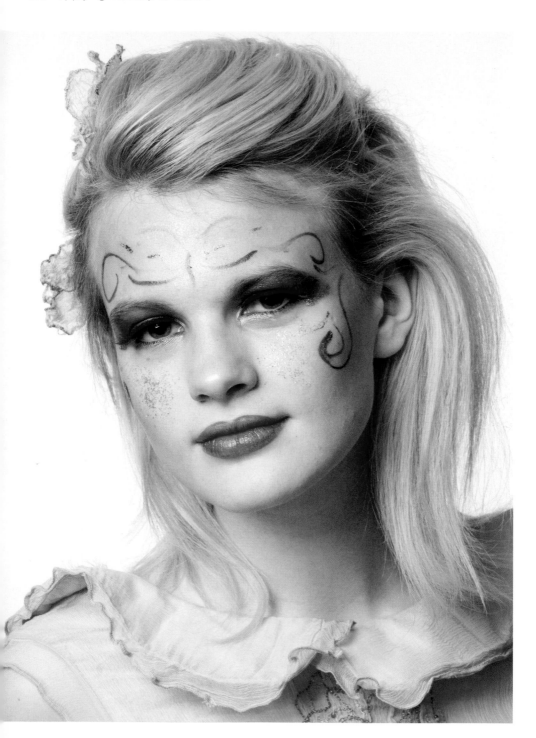

Costume party casualty

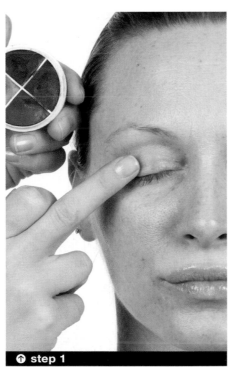

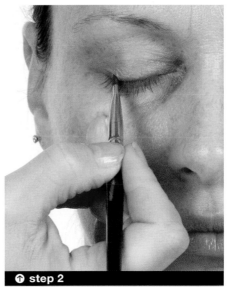

⬆ step 2

Apply purple greasepaint to the inner corner and on the lower socket to create a shadow. Work along the lash line with a detail or lip brush.

⬆ step 1

To create a black eye, apply yellow/green greasepaint from a bruise wheel over the whole eye area.

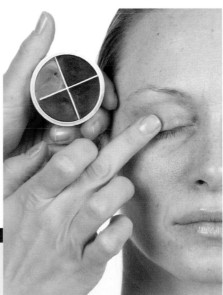

➔ step 3

Smudge in using your finger.

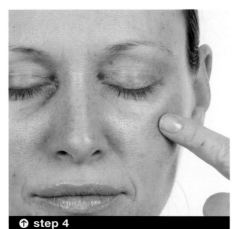

⬆ step 4

Create a bruised cheek by smudging green over the cheek.

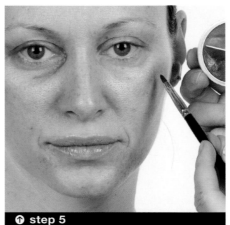

⬆ step 5

Add purple and blue/black to the center of the cheekbone. Dot the paint on using a brush, and smudge it in with your little finger. Lightly press loose powder over the greasepaint to set and prevent it from creasing.

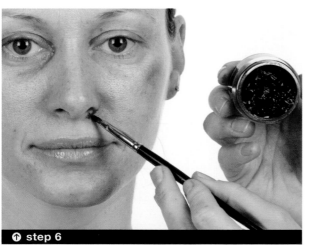

⬆ step 6

Darken around one nostril with purple greasepaint and add some fake blood.

Pro Tip

To vary the intensity of this makeup, you can play with the amount of bruising and blood that you use.

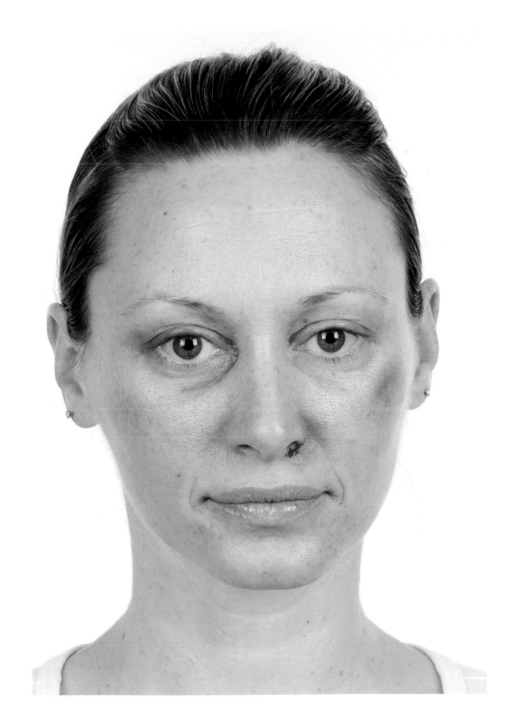

Costume party casualty

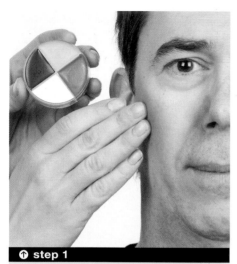

↑ step 1

Apply red greasepaint to the cheek, over one eye, and around the nose.

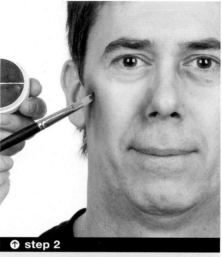

↑ step 2

Darken the central area of red with a darker hue.

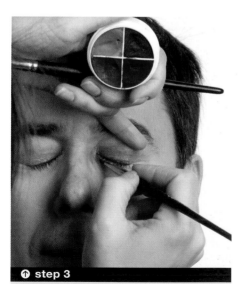

↑ step 3

Darken the inner corner of the eye and along the bottom and top lash lines.

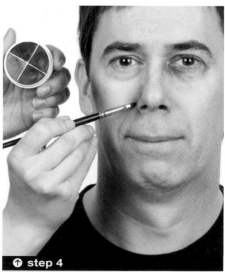

↑ step 4

Add fake blood.

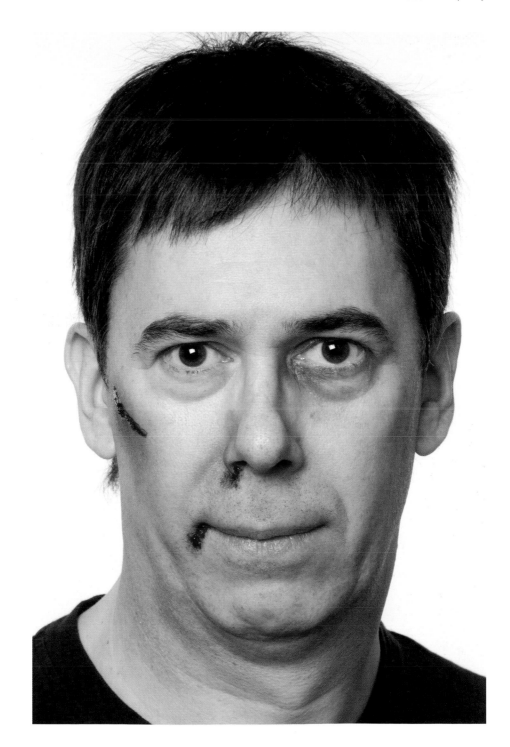

Costume party 1960s

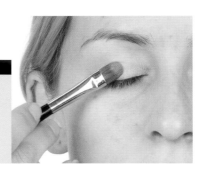

➔ step 1

Prepare skin. Starting with the eyes, use a nude base (cream eye color or foundation) all over. Press pale matte pink (or white) eyeshadow onto the inner half of the eyelid and over the high point.

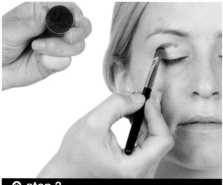

↑ step 2

Start to build the socket, adding a little at a time, using a matte black or very dark gray. Shade the outer half of the lid, along the socket and slightly onto the upper part of the lid, for a theatrical effect.

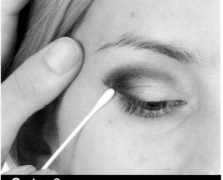

↑ step 3

Lift the outer corner of the shading upward so that when the eye is open, it gives a slightly flicked effect. Alternatively, once shading is finished, clean with a cotton swab at the corner of the eye to give a flicked effect.

➔ step 4

With a kohl pencil, line along the top lashes, close to the lash line and inside the lower eye. Blend well to soften all hard edges. Groom the brows and lightly fill in if necessary—they should not be heavy.

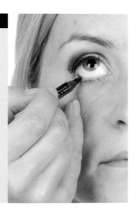

➔ step 5

Curl the lashes and add a thin coat of mascara. Apply a full set of false eyelashes on top.

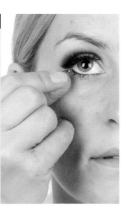

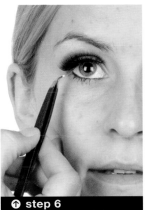

↳ step 7

To contour the cheeks, shade under the cheekbones with beige or skin-color blush that is two shades darker than the skin tone.

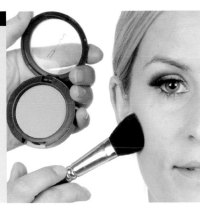

↑ step 6

Lightly apply a second coat of mascara to the false and real lashes, to emphasize them and combine them together.

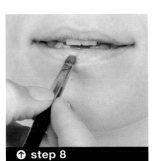

↑ step 8

Apply frosted pink lipstick—no need for lipliner. Powder lightly to set.

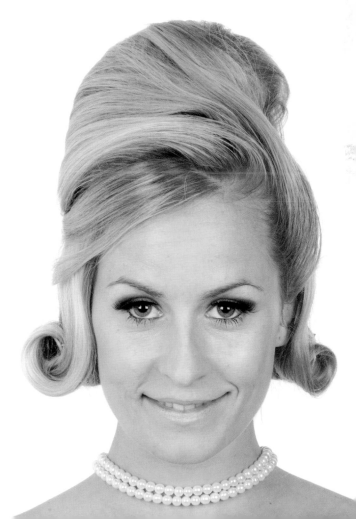

Costume party Regency

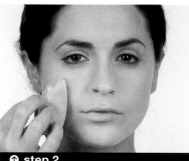

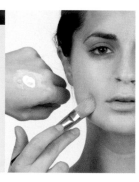

● step 1

Apply a pale liquid base using a foundation brush— you could try mixing white into your palest foundation to achieve the correct color.

⬆ step 2

Set with translucent white powder, using a velour puff. Press the puff against the face and roll the powder into the skin, repeating until it disappears.

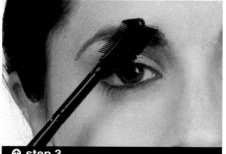

⬆ step 3

Groom the eyebrows with a wand and define their arched shape with an eyebrow pencil, but do not add any width—Georgian women preferred very thin eyebrows.

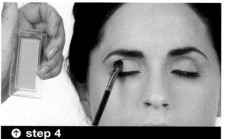

⬆ step 4

Prepare the eye area by applying foundation over the eyelid and setting with translucent powder. Give the eye shape and depth by shading the socket with a taupe eyeshadow.

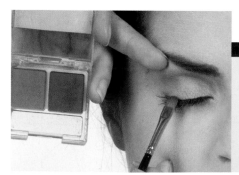

⬅ step 5

Define the eye by lining around the lash line on the top and bottom lids with a matte brown eyeshadow, lifting the brow to get to the root of the lashes.

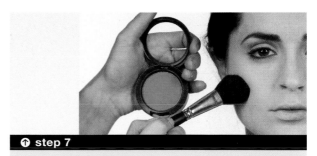

↑ step 6

Draw on a lip line with a nude lip pencil to obtain the correct shape. Start with the bow, drawing inward one side at a time, making it neat and rounded. Draw in the outer edges from the outside inward so the line is solid. Draw the lips narrower than they really are, so they appear fuller. Repeat on the bottom lip. When the lipline is correct, go over it with a red pencil and fill in with lipstick. Blot for a matte finish.

↑ step 7

Apply a red-based blusher sparingly with a blusher brush—circle it on just below the apples of the cheeks. Georgian women wore rouge in a rounded shape quite low down the cheek.

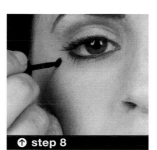

↑ step 8

Replicate a Georgian face patch—used to cover blemishes or marks—using liquid eyeliner. Here it is worn close to the eye and looks much like a beauty spot.

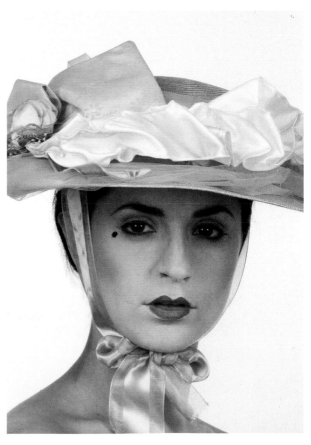

Costume party eighteenth century

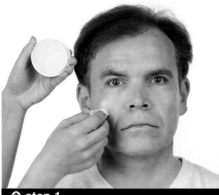

↑ step 1

Apply a base in a pale tone (but not white) all over the face, including the eyelids. Use either a cream foundation applied with a foundation brush and blended with fingers, or an aqua color applied with a damp sponge and worked quickly into the skin.

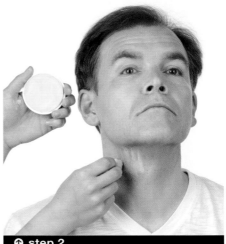

↑ step 2

Continue the application of base down over the neck and ears.

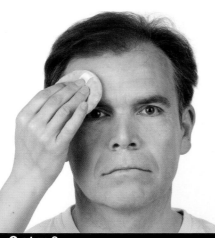

↑ step 3

Set with loose transculent powder. Press the powder into the skin using a velour puff and work it in until the powder disappears.

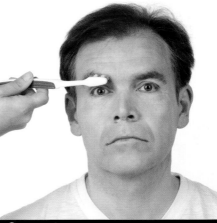

↑ step 4

Groom the eyebrows with a toothbrush and brush the hairs on the inner half upward and those toward the outside downward to exaggerate the arch. Set with brow gel or by spraying a little hairspray onto your fingers and smoothing over.

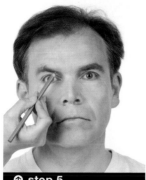

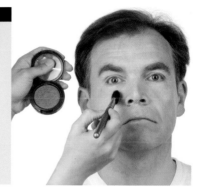

➔ step 6

Apply a small amount of blush in a rust tone, circling it over the apples of the cheeks, and blending downward along the sides of the nose.

↑ step 5

To strengthen the brow further, you can lightly pencil through with an eyebrow pencil.

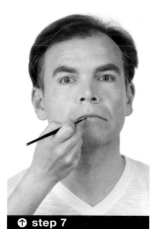

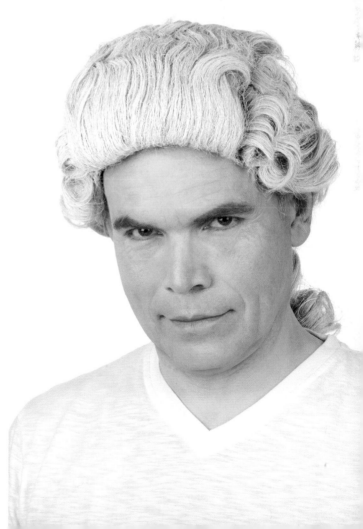

↑ step 7

Smudge a small amount of matte brown-red lipstick onto the lips with a lip brush. Work it well into the lips and blot. It should just look like a wash of color.

Costume party Wild West

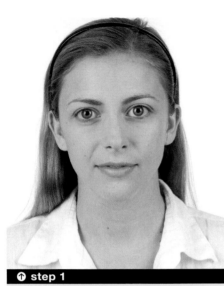

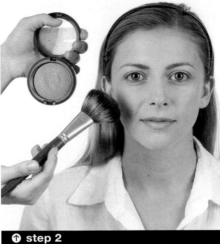

↑ step 2

Apply a golden shade of bronzer on the high points of the face, where the sun naturally colors the skin—across the top of the nose, on the apples of the cheeks, and on the forehead and chin.

↑ step 1

Apply a base all over the face, using a tinted moisturizer in a warm shade. Use concealer where necessary. Lightly set with loose powder on the T-zone.

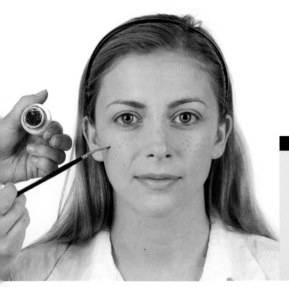

← step 3

Add freckles to the cheeks and the bridge of the nose, using a soft brown eyeliner pencil or kohl from a pot with a fine detail brush.

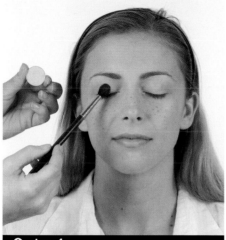

⬆ step 4

Prepare the eye area with a nude beige powder or cream eyeshadow. Apply from the lash line to the brow, to neutralize the color of the eye and absorb any excess oil.

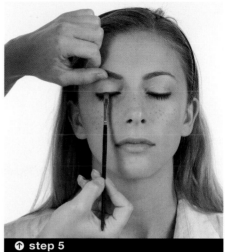

⬆ step 5

Groom the eyebrows. There is no need to darken them or add volume for this look. Apply brown eyeliner along the upper lash line using a kohl pencil. Work from the outer edge inward, and then back out toward the outer edge. Work over the line with a detail brush to ensure you have a solid, unbroken line.

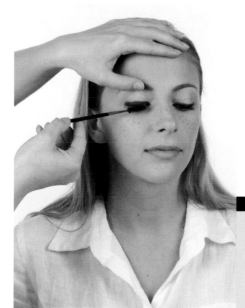

⬅ step 6

Curl the eyelashes and apply one coat of mascara.

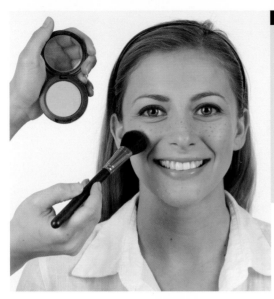

⬅ step 7

Apply a rose-pink blush to the apples of the cheeks. Lightly touch the brush into the product and dab onto the apples, building up the application a little at a time.

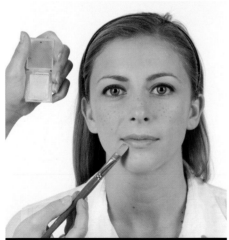

⬆ step 8

To enhance and define the natural lip line, work around the edge of the mouth, outside of the lip line, using a concealer slightly lighter than the skin, and blend outward.

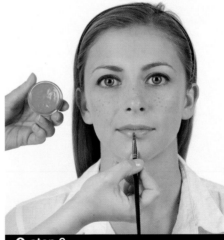

⬆ step 9

Draw on the lip line using a light pink lip pencil, then fill in the whole lip area with the same pencil. Add lip gloss on top. To finish, lightly powder the whole face with a loose, translucent powder.

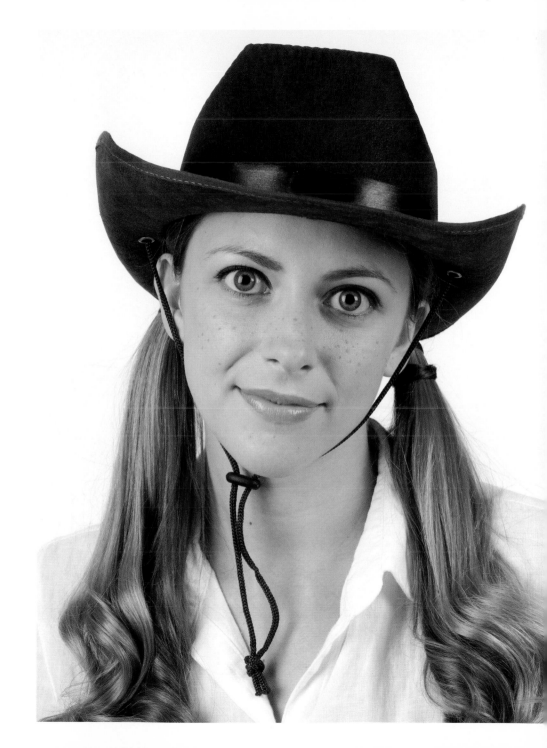

Costume party 1930s

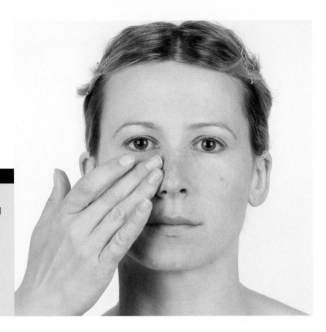

➔ step 1

Cleanse the skin and apply a base all over the face, including the eyelids. Use a concealer where necessary.

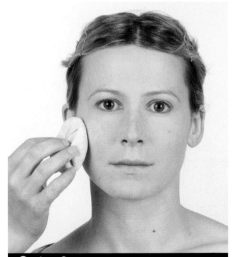

⬆ step 2

Powder to set, using translucent powder. Roll the powder onto the skin using a velour puff, then dust away the excess with a powder brush.

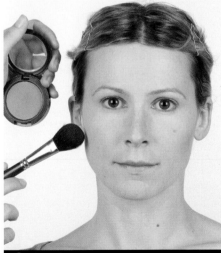

⬆ step 3

Apply a dark-tone contouring blush beneath the cheekbones.

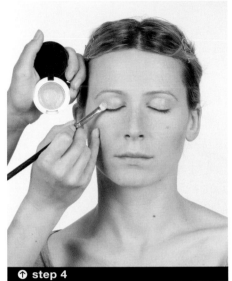

↑ step 4

Use a pearly blue eyeshadow to highlight the eyelids.

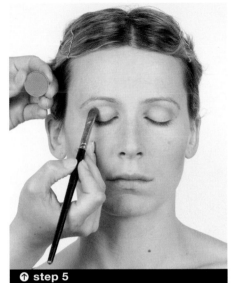

↑ step 5

Enhance the socket line with lilac eyeshadow. Apply the eyeshadow using a large eyeshadow brush, and blend well.

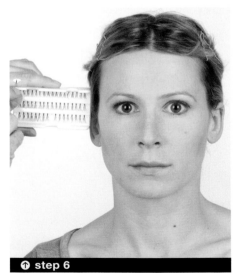

↑ step 6

Apply some sections of false eyelashes (see page 94).

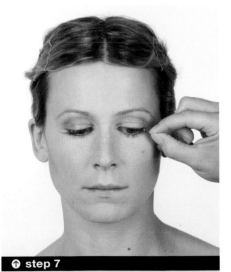

↑ step 7

Focus the length of the added lashes on the outside of the upper lids. Apply mascara.

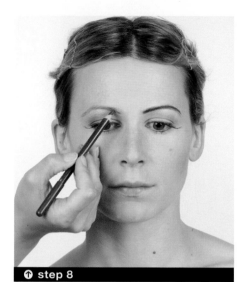

⬆ step 8

Enhance the shape of the eyebrows using a sharpened brown eyebrow pencil. Work from the inner edge of the brow outward, drawing with the pencil in short strokes, to mimic hairs.

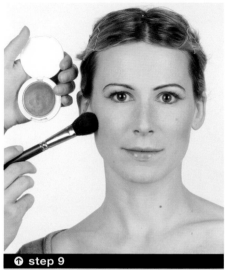

⬆ step 9

Apply a dusky rose cream blush from the apples, back toward the ears.

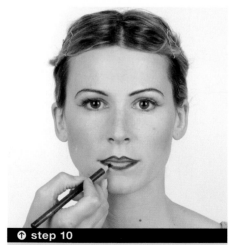

⬆ step 10

Line the lips so they look full, with a pronounced bow (see page 82).

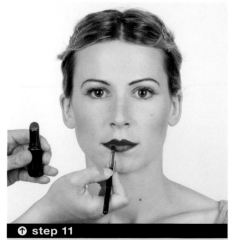

⬆ step 11

Fill in the lip area with lipstick, blot, and repeat.

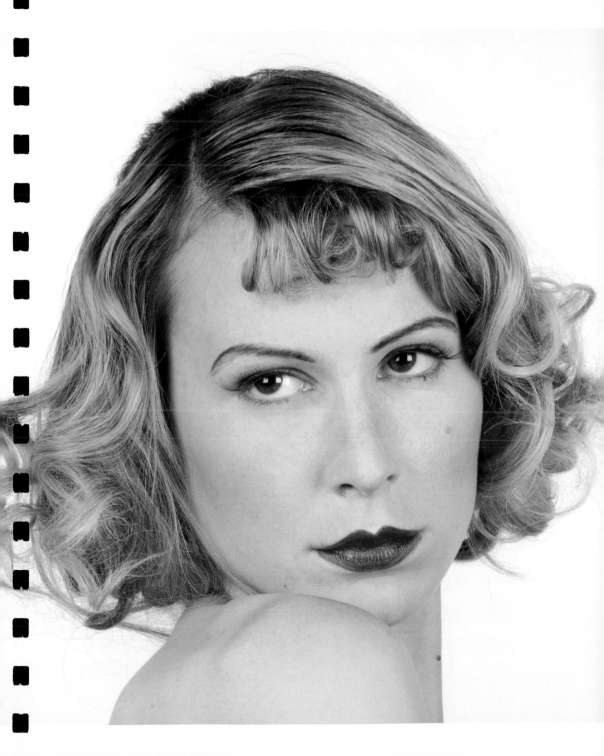

Costume party 1930s

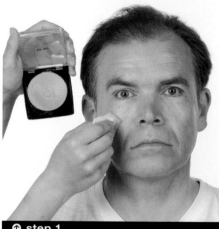

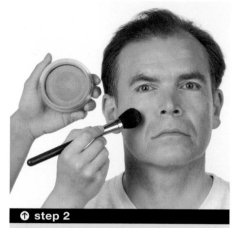

↑ step 1

Following the makeup for men routine (see pages 200–1), use a wash of cake makeup over the whole face, including the eyes, and conceal where necessary. Look for redness around the eyes and nostrils.

↑ step 2

Add a matte cream bronzer on the high points of the face (cheeks, bridge of nose, forehead) and then powder to set. If you have a powder blush, powder first and then lightly dust with the bronzer. Ensure the bronzer is matte and contains no shimmer.

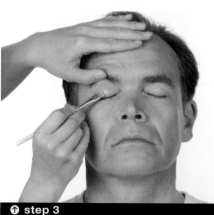

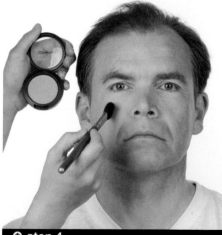

↑ step 3

Add a small highlight to the high point of the eyelid to open the eye up. Use base or a small amount of concealer in a shade paler than that of the foundation.

↑ step 4

Apply a small amount of a matte peachy blush on either side of the nose in an upside-down triangular shape.

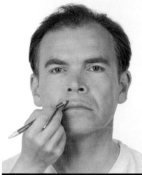

⬆ step 5

The mustache is small and neat as an alternative to laying on a crepe hair mustache. Draw it on with an eyebrow pencil. Starting with a light pencil, draw small hairs by making downward strokes, starting in the middle and working toward the outside.

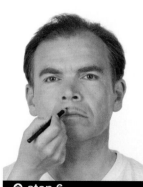

⬆ step 6

Fill in darker hairs sporadically with a darker pencil.

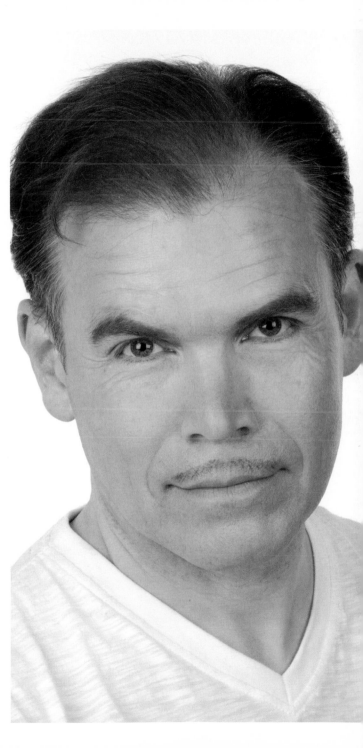

Costume party 1940s

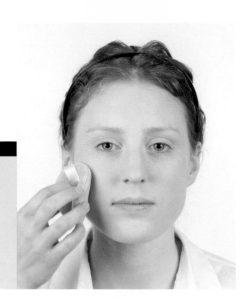

● step 1

Prepare the skin; apply a matte base of normal to heavy coverage, and conceal where necessary. Dust with powder to set. Roll on with a puff until the powder disappears into the skin.

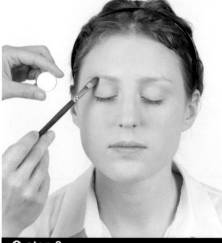

⬆ step 2

Prepare the eye area, using foundation all over the lid up to the brow. Apply a nude beige eyeshadow over the whole lid, highlighting under the arch of the brow with a matte white eyeshadow.

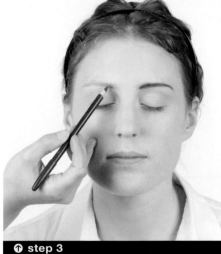

⬆ step 3

Enhance the eyebrows, using a dark brown pencil and working in small strokes.

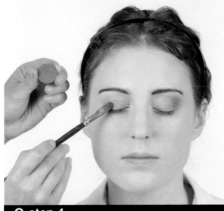

⬆ step 4

Using a matte, muted pale gray, apply eyeshadow from the lash line over the whole lid, up to the socket line. Blend the shadow up toward the brow on the outer half of the eye only. Blend well to soften the edges.

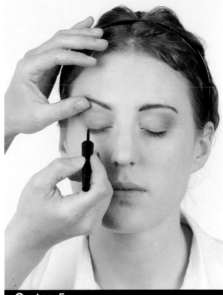

⬆ step 5

Using liquid eyeliner, draw a line along the top lashes, as close to the root of the lashes as you can get. To help you to reach right to the root of the lashes, lift the top lid gently by placing your thumb under the brow. Under the eyes should be left clean.

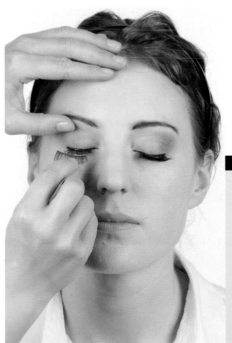

⬅ step 6

Curl the eyelashes and apply mascara to both top and bottom (this blends into the false eyelashes better). Apply a full set of false eyelashes (see page 95).

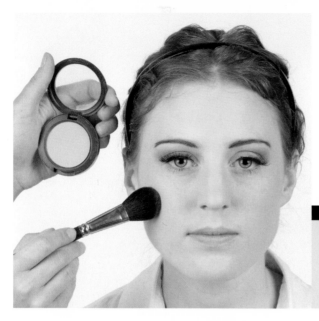

← step 7

Apply a rosy powder blush slightly beneath the cheekbone.

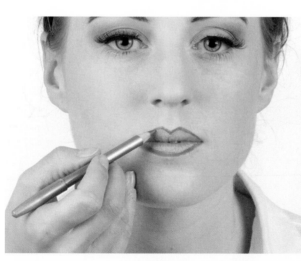

← step 8

Draw in the lip line slightly outside of the lips using a pencil lipliner (line first with nude so that it is easier to correct if you make a mistake). Fill in with lip pencil to create a lip base. Coat with a red lipstick (use one with a pinky, rather than an orangey, base), blot, and apply lip gloss.

Pro tip

When applying blusher, do so after powdering if you are using a powdered blush, and before powdering if using a cream blush so that the powder helps it to set.

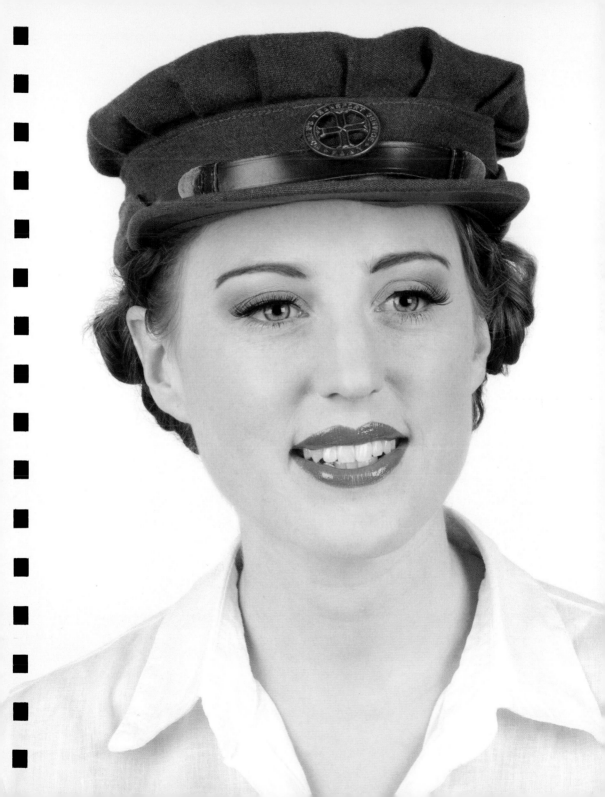

Costume party Renaissance

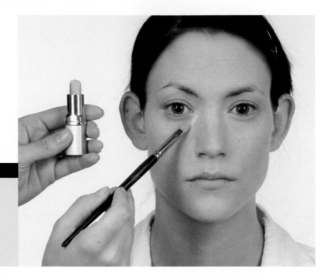

→ step 1

Prepare the skin, applying a base as described on page 46. Use a light foundation in a pale shade.

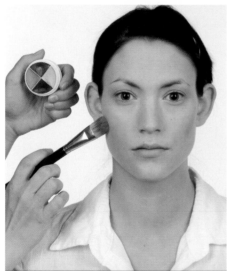

↑ step 2

Apply concealer with a concealer brush where required (see page 50). Blend into the foundation with your finger.

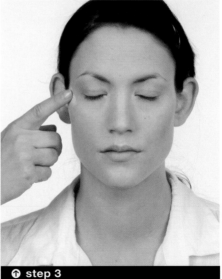

↑ step 3

Shade and highlight the face (see page 60) to improve the bone structure.

➔ step 4

Groom the eyebrows by combing through. Fill in the brows if necessary with brow powder in a shade compatible with the natural color of the hairs. Use a slanted eyebrow brush and start at the inner corner. With small strokes of the brush, work outward over the arch to the outer edge.

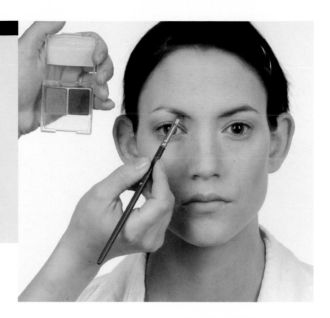

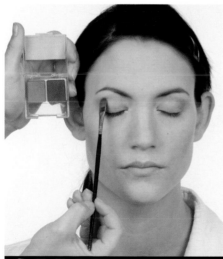

⬆ step 5

Give the eyes depth by shading the socket line with a matte brown eyeshadow. Apply a little shadow at a time and blend well so no hard lines are visible.

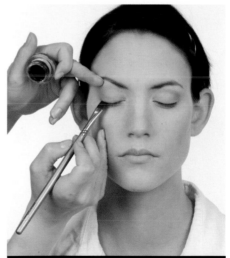

⬆ step 6

Enhance the eyes by applying a dark brown or black kohl eyeliner close to the lashes on the top lids only. Curl the eyelashes and apply mascara.

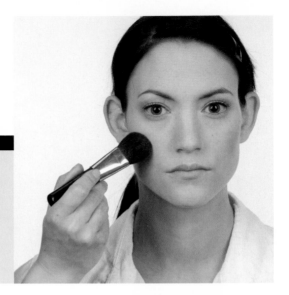

➔ step 7

Italian women in the Renaissance often wore rouge circled heavily around the apples of their cheeks, but this look is slightly more subtle. Choose a reddish pink tone and apply lightly, swirling over the apples.

➔ step 8

Apply a burned-red lip stain by dabbing lipstick onto the lips with your finger and blotting. This will give a natural finish.

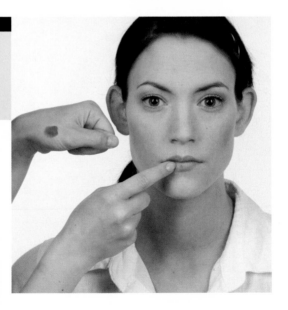

Pro Tip

If you don't have blush in the right tone, use a dab of lipstick in the appropriate shade and work it into the skin with your fingers.

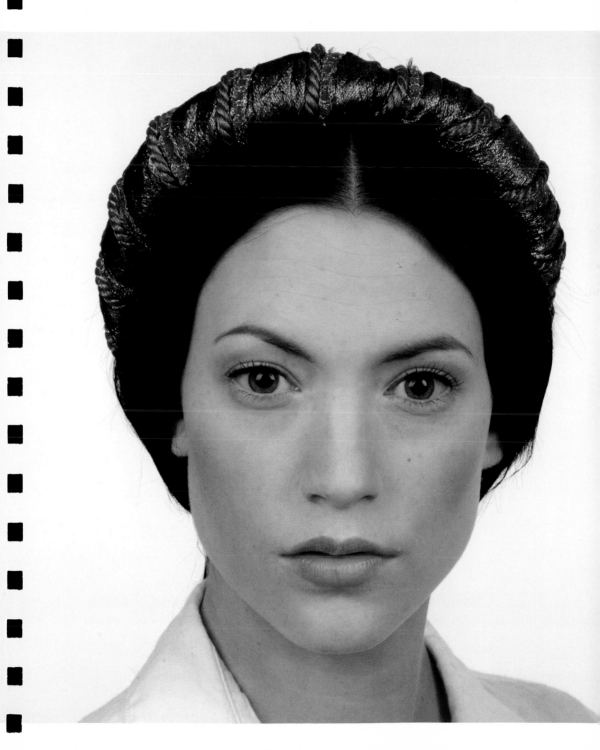

Costume party Gothic

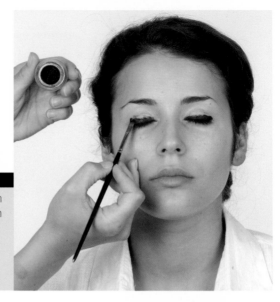

Smudge black eyeliner along the top lash line using either a pencil or a kohl liner in a pot with a flat liner brush.

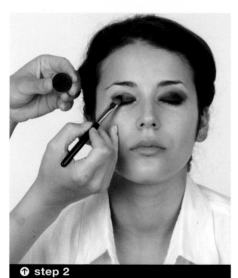

⬆ step 2

Brush a matte black eyeshadow over the eyeliner and smudge up toward the socket, blending the edges so the color fades away.

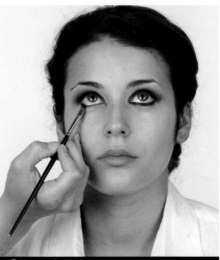

⬆ step 3

Use a fine detail brush to line the lower eyelid close to the lash line.

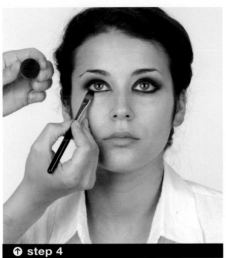

⬆ step 4

Ask your model to look away as you line around the eyes.

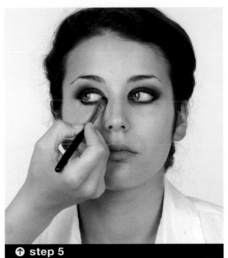

⬆ step 5

Smudge the eyeshadow under the eyes with a clean brush.

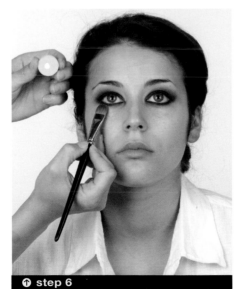

⬆ step 6

Blend in a nude matte beige eyeshadow just below the black eyeliner.

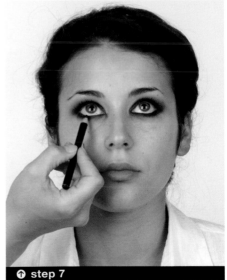

⬆ step 7

Apply eyeliner to the inside of the lower eyelid with a black kohl pencil.

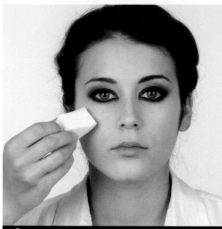

↑ step 8

Clean the skin to remove any fallen eyeshadow. Use a foundation sponge to apply a pale foundation mixed with a small amount of white greasepaint.

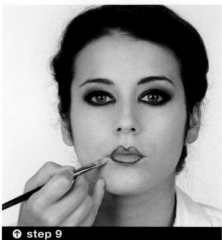

↑ step 9

Block out the corners of the lips with a very pale foundation or concealer. Powder, then draw the outline of a full, bow-shaped lip (see page 82).

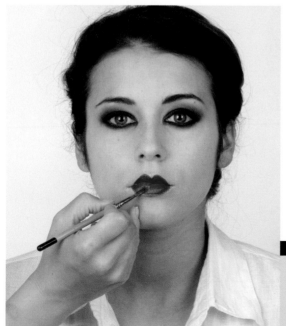

↩ step 10

Fill in the lips with lipstick, using a lip brush, and blot and repeat.

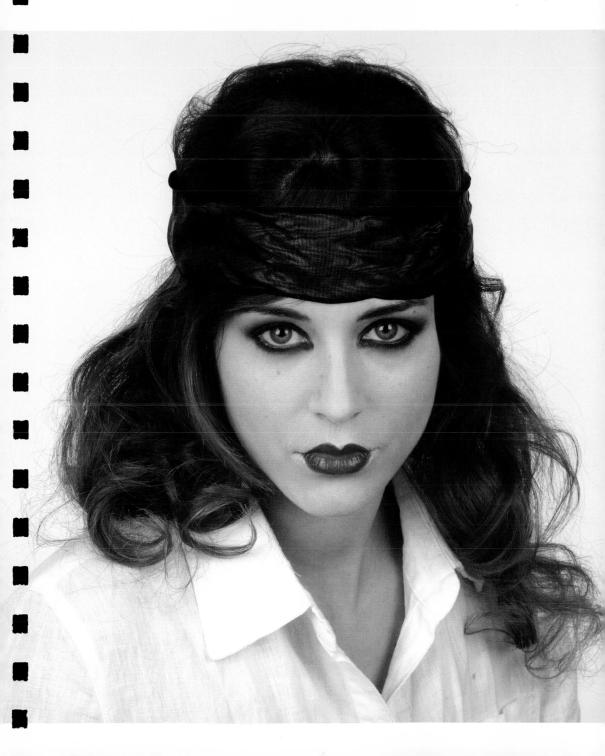

TAKING IT FURTHER

Makeup is a very rewarding career. I really enjoy working for myself, having no two weeks the same, and constantly meeting and working with new people. It is equally exciting to work on a live TV show that will be watched by millions of people, to create an image for a photo shoot, or to be part of a bride's big day.

Makeup artists can work with individual, private clients and brides, as well as in theater, TV, film, advertising, special effects, and the music or publishing industries. Some people specialize in one area and develop very specific skills, while others work simultaneously in many aspects of makeup to keep their skills very broad.

To be a makeup artist, it is essential to get some formal training. This can range from intensive short courses to two or three years of full-time study. The type of training you choose is likely to depend on your age, what aspect of makeup you want to work in, and what skills you already have. Some courses can be expensive, so I recommend you do some research before making a choice. Ask to see the resumes and work of past students and lecturers; make sure the pupils have gone on to work in the areas you are interested in; and confirm that the people who will be teaching you have had successful careers themselves.

After taking courses, your next step is to assist an established artist. This will be for little or no pay, but it is essential to learn etiquette skills for working on a set as well as the practical aspects of the job that can't be taught in the classroom.

A makeup artist needs a portfolio of work and a showreel to send to potential clients. Portfolios are developed on test shoots where a makeup artist will get together with a photographer, stylist, and model, who are also building their portfolios. Everyone is working for free and costs may be split. Short films are good for making film contacts and building a showreel (lots of film school students make short films during weekends).

If you are thinking about a career in makeup, practice doing makeup on as many faces as possible. This is the best way to get a feel for what does and doesn't work on different face shapes, skin tones, and ages. When I started my freelance career, I also worked in a makeup shop, which was a great way to learn about different products and practice on different faces.

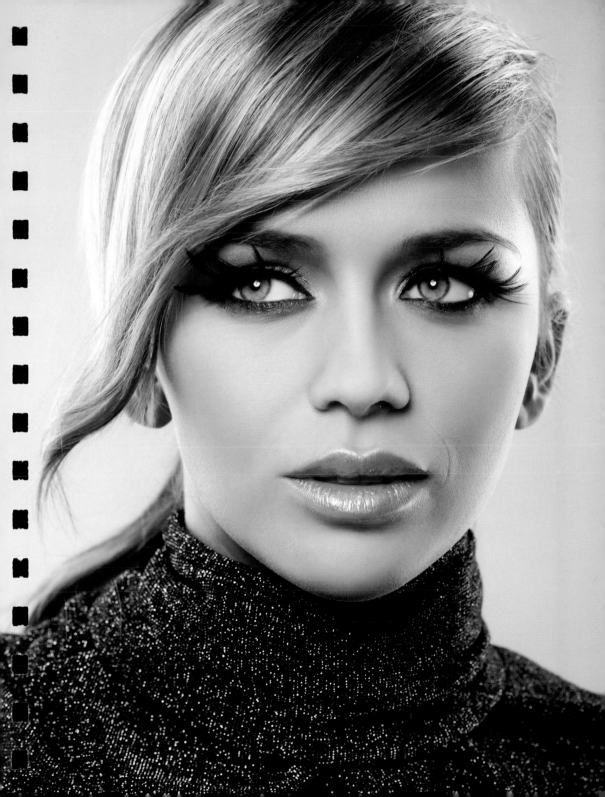

SUPPLIERS

Makeup

www.maccosmetics.com
www.narscosmetics.com
www.shuuemura.com
www.dior.com
www.chanel.com
www.shiseido.com
www.makeupforever.com
www.chantecaille.com
www.clinique.com
www.maxfactor.com
www.fresh.com
www.byterry.com
www.loreal.com
www.maybelline.com
www.urbandecay.com
www.cargocosmetics.com
www.loraccosmetics.com

Specialist treatment/ camouflage makeup

www.dremablend.com
www.coverfx.com

Skincare

www.dermalogica.com

Tools

www.japonesque.com
www.tweezerman.com

Special effects/ face painting

www.bennye.com
www.kryolan.com

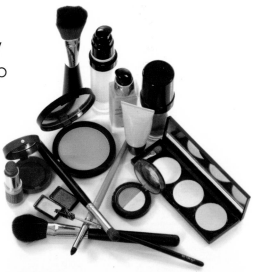

CREDITS

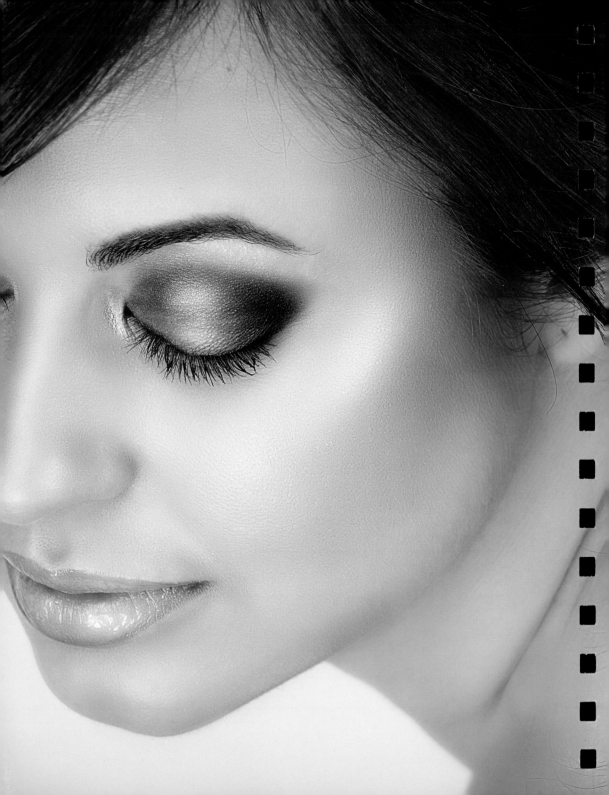

INDEX

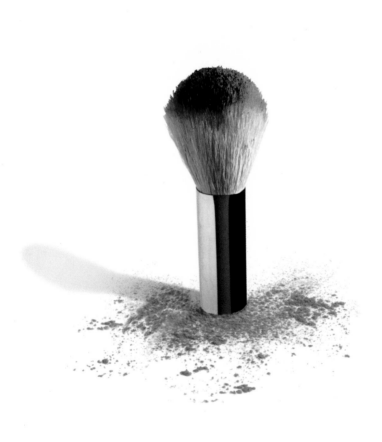